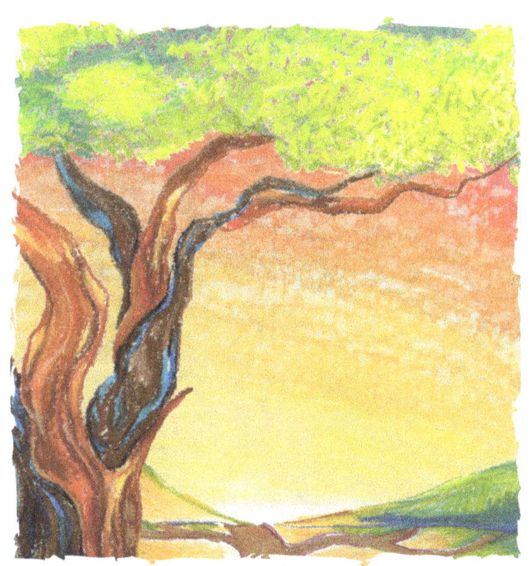

COLORED PAPERS UNDER
THE ACACIA TREE

About the Authors

Michelle Hinton Larsen lives in Utah, USA, and has been passionate about women's health since her first university class in 1990. Michelle has a Masters degree in Health Education and feels especially called to help all people understand the benefits of revering, understanding, and protecting the body and soul. She works as a philanthropist, mother to nine children, author, business owner, and wife.

Emily Motsi, based in Nairobi, Kenya, is a certified counseling psychologist and an expert in technology and customer service. With a passion for continuous learning and personal growth, she combines her diverse expertise to provide exceptional support and innovative solutions. Emily is also an avid traveler, keen on exploring new cultures and destinations.

Kelsey Evans is a Denver, CO based designer and illustrator. She is passionate about creating and using art as a way to tell meaningful stories. In her work, she likes using color and texture to express emotion, movement, and spirit. She finds her inspiration in nature and experiencing different creative cultures around the world.

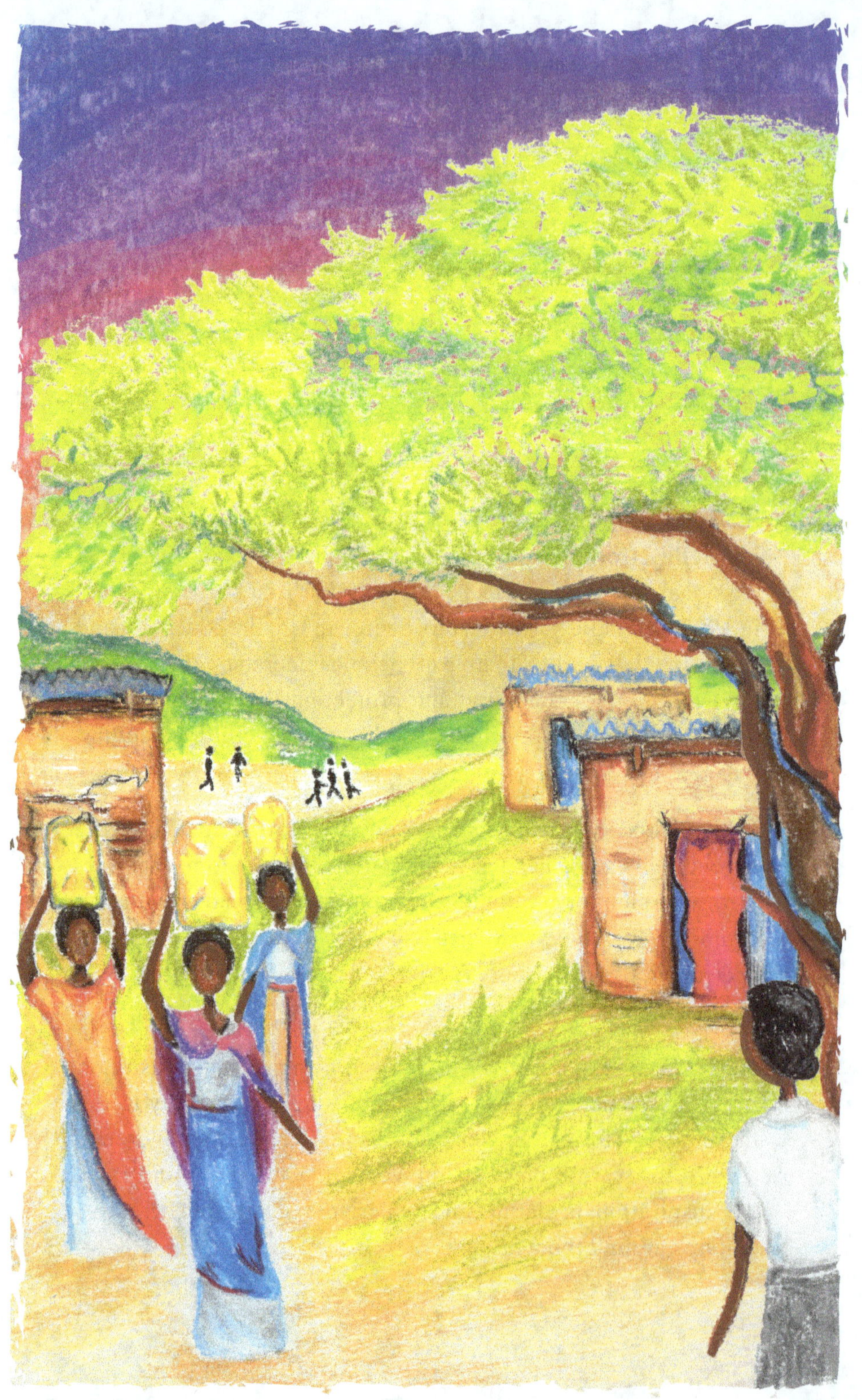

Chapter One

The sunset cast a warm orange glow over the expansive savannah and dusty paths came alive with tired footfalls, signaling the end of another day. Pendo noticed how poverty carved life's challenges on the faces of Ubora's African residents in her village.

At the center of the settlement stood a cluster of mud homes with worn thatched roofs after years of rain. Despite their appearance, they had a sense of warmth. The air smelled of basic meals made with gathered or traded items while cooking fires smoked.

Boys laughed and played with makeshift soccer balls crafted from plastic bags and twine. Some wore shoes patched together with scraps of leather, however, no one seemed to care. Amid their sufferings, their laughter was a symphony. One youngster made a toy car from tin cans, symbolizing a spirit of optimism and resourcefulness that prevailed where only a handful could afford transportation beyond their own two feet.

Women wearing bright kanga clothes and torn t-shirts gathered around a nearby well. They carefully carried fresh water home in huge yellow plastic cans on their heads. They laughed and encouraged each other with chit-chat of the day.

After a long day of walking to and from school, the task of fetching water weighed heavily on Pendo. She occupied her mind with her demanding studies and maneuvered the cumbersome water can with determination. Her focus was unwavering as she aimed to complete her tasks swiftly, hoping to allocate some time for her readings before nightfall. Pendo was too focused on heaving the water canister to notice the blood that stained her thin school uniform and was now running down her leg.

The water can fell off her head as she lost her concentration. Sighing in frustration, Pendo felt the world's weight on her shoulders. She had not prepared for this month's menstruation cycle and was caught off guard by its sudden arrival. Fortunately, she had been near home back when she had started her first cycle. With a stroke of luck, she had found scraps of old fabric to use as a makeshift pad. Her mother had gently asked her father for money to buy disposable sanitary pads, understanding the importance of proper hygiene during menstruation. Her father, burdened by the family's financial struggles, grumbled that it was time Pendo provided for herself.

This time, there were no scraps of fabric. She would have to pass by the group of boys playing football, and that would be the beginning of endless taunts and jeers, a torment that had already driven many of her friends to drop out of the seventh grade. A girl can only finish school if she has access to sanitary supplies. If the four days of absence fell on an exam day or when an exam review happened, she most likely could not pass her exams. Since no twelve-year-old girl could afford the pads independently, that led to only one outcome: few girls were graduating from the eighth grade in the village.

The only girls who could continue attending school after they began menstruating were those fortunate enough to have supportive parents who could buy them sanitary pads. Unfortunately, Pendo's parents could not afford such things. As she felt the trickle of blood down her legs, a wave of despair threatened and tears welled up in her eyes. She refused to let them fall as this would only fuel the fire of remarks from the boys. Extreme sorrow swelled in her heart as she foresaw her own fate.

Suddenly, she felt a sweater wrapped around her waist. She quietly turned to see that Maryam, an acquaintance a few years older, had rescued her in the nick of time. Maryam walked behind her nonchalantly, her water jug sloshing on her head.

Pendo stopped abruptly, eyes widening in disbelief. The sweater felt like a shield, sparing her from the fate of becoming a day laborer, at least for another month. Maryam silently urged Pendo forward with a glance as if they were strangers passing by on the street.

Maryam's attention shifted back to Pendo after she realized they had passed the group of football players. With a radiant smile, Maryam approached Pendo as if they had been friends for years.

Still trying to make sense of the chaotic sequence of events, Pendo hesitated. Her emotions were all over her face. Trembling, she introduced herself. "Hi! I'm Pendo."

"I saw you and knew I had to help." Maryam's words held genuine warmth. "No one needs to know what time of the month it is." They laughed nervously, knowing that being shamed for a period accident could have extreme effects on a girl's future.

Pendo felt a knot in her throat as she thought of Maryam's bravery and kindness. She choked out a grateful, "Thank you," eyes shining with emotion.

The next day, Maryam brought a few of her menstrual supplies and placed them in Pendo's care. "Keep these with you at all times."

They became friends quickly. Maryam's fearlessness inspired Pendo to be adventurous, while Pendo's cautiousness kept Maryam from overstepping her boundaries. They met daily on their long walks to the village center. Pendo's timidity dissolved through their many conversations as Maryam's words of encouragement urged her to speak her mind on many topics. Pendo admired Maryam's sense of adventure and bravery despite village hardships. In turn, Maryam sensed a calm strength and gentle heart beyond Pendo's shy, quiet nature.

In the humble surroundings of the village, where hardship was as common as the dusty paths that crisscrossed the settlement, Maryam and Pendo found comfort in each other. They exchanged future dreams and current challenges at the same water stream that had started their bond.

One afternoon, as they walked along the outskirts of the settlement, Maryam looked at Pendo with a cryptic grin and a gleam of joy in her eyes. "Pendo, have you heard about the professional doctor woman who visits the village clinic every month?"

Pendo nodded. "Yes. I overheard my aunties talking of her. They say she provides medicine to treat infections of our private areas and help us understand why we burn, itch, and hurt when we relieve ourselves."

Maryam's face lit up. "Yes! Rumor has it that this miracle

worker will be returning to our community later today. It seems like we need to visit her. She can probably advise us on so many of the topics we have discussed." She leaned close. "All the things we do not dare to ask our mothers."

Pendo was hesitant since her shy personality made her nervous in social situations. "What's the point of meeting her?" Her voice was tinged with uncertainty. "We have our aunties to learn from. It is tradition to ask them first."

Maryam's eyes lit with enthusiasm. "True. Our aunties and mothers are our elders and they are wise, and I respect them deeply. This woman was educated in science while also having our cultural values and upbringing. And not only that but she was educated with the men folk! I wonder how she had the money, the time away from her obligations and chores, and the bravery to become a doctor. She surely had to go to school in the city surrounded by strangers. She will have some fresh and new perspectives different from what we know."

Pendo seriously thought about what Maryam said and realized she was right. She was excited and daunted by the prospect of hearing how she cured so many illnesses—cures that might go against their village traditions. "What if what she says goes against what older people have taught us?" Pendo's voice held a note of doubt.

Maryam extended a comforting hand to rest on Pendo's shoulder, her reassuring touch grounding her fears. "Then we will consider it. We have our own minds, our own lives, and we get to decide. Someone has to be right. Right?"

"Okay, Maryam. Let's go meet her," Pendo said.

Invigorated by the prospect of new knowledge and possibilities,

Maryam smiled with excitement. "Great! I knew you'd agree. Come on, let's head to the clinic before she arrives."

As they made their way to the clinic, they crossed paths with Nyah and Farida. Nyah, a beautiful and hard-working girl who they knew from their church congregation and Farida, her cousin. They saw them often and they had both shared an all-too-common fate awaiting them. Nyah's dreams of becoming a teacher were overshadowed by her family's insistence on an early marriage. It was a common and long-standing tradition, so much so that most girls do not dream of anything more than to be given to a man in exchange for a dowry to be paid to their family. This tradition is so embedded into culture that it is what a family counts on for economic gain. Farida, with her quiet strength, had undergone Female Genital Mutilation and carried the emotional scars of that experience.

Maryam, noticing the apprehension on their faces, approached them with a gentle smile. "We're heading to the clinic to meet Dr. Emma. She's a professional doctor who visits our village every month. We are going to meet with her to ask questions. Would you like to join us?"

Nyah and Farida exchanged glances, their curiosity piqued. "Do you think she can teach us?" Nyah asked, her voice tinged with hope and uncertainty.

"I believe so," Maryam replied confidently. "She has had more schooling than anyone else we know. She must know something."

With a newfound sense of hope, Nyah and Farida joined Maryam and Pendo on their journey to the clinic.

Chapter Two

-----

*A*s they watched the doctor from afar, the four girls were captivated by her aura of knowledge and authority. They wondered at her commanding, yet gentle, voice. At first glance, no one would think she was anything special. To see her in her doctor's coat relating to people and listening to her speak of how they each had the power to save their own lives, this Dr. Emma seemed larger than life. Stories of her wisdom and ability to connect the old ways with modern practices had given her a reputation that spread like wildfire through the surrounding villages.

Waiting until she finished with her patients, they approached Dr. Emma as she sat beside a tall acacia tree behind the clinic, slicing a mango with a small knife. Her presence was both charming and reassuring. She peacefully smiled and greeted them. "Hello. I'm Dr. Emma."

Maryam, Pendo, Nyah, and Farida introduced themselves. Pendo tried not to let her awe and interest overcome her. After weeks of being around Maryam's courageous spirit, Pendo spoke up. "Dr. Emma, we've heard of your knowledge of the body and how to be healthy in our traditions and with modern life. We want to learn and understand this too!"

Dr. Emma's quiet voice felt reassuring. "Of course. I want nothing more than to help young women like you. You are the hope of our future world. Even now, this community needs you to understand yourselves, love yourselves, and then give all that understanding and love to others. That is not a new idea." She chuckled. "But I would also like very much to teach you facts that will open up amazing possibilities."

Dr. Emma knew very well the severity of the health threats facing these girls and worried often about facts of health inside the restraints of their culture. She had witnessed it too often in the bodies and minds of her patients as she traveled through the villages. Dr. Emma wanted to lead them on a journey of health that included mind, body, and spirit. As they met each week, she introduced them to the importance of being healthy, happy, and holy. She spoke of the balance in nature and within themselves, emphasizing the importance of cherishing their bodies as vessels for their precious minds and souls.

Finally, the day came when she had ample time and the village was healthy during her weekly visit. She gathered the girls and began to teach on the importance of making healthy decisions.

"I understand healthy and not healthy as far as my body feeling sick," Pendo said. "What do you mean when you say my decisions affect the health of my mind or soul?"

Dr. Emma smiled gently, knowing this was a crucial question. "Every part of us—body, mind, and soul—is interconnected. Our choices affect not just our physical health but also our mental and spiritual well-being. I grew up not far from here. In my village, girls had no say in whom they married or when they were to be married. For many of the families, it was customary to make a financial arrangement for the marriage of their daughters. It led to a mindset for girls to only think of themselves as property." The doctor sighed and looked up to the cloudless sky where the sun found no relief.

"Many of my young friends were given in marriage before they were mature enough to carry children. Many were abused and made to work tirelessly. Of course, the young developing body of the girl was not considered in these transactions, let alone the mind or soul. Many of these girls died early because their bodies were too young to bear children. Some families, however, saw the error in this tradition. Thankfully, mine was one such family.

My mother entered marriage at a young age. She boldly decided to alter our family's future by reshaping her beliefs. With determination, she sang to me as she braided my hair, "Healthy am I. Happy am I. Holy am I." Those words were ingrained in my soul and became my motto. I would say those words as others around me wanted to treat me as property. When many of my friends engaged in irresponsible sexual behaviors, I would say these words. When someone ridiculed me for focusing on school over boys, I would say those words. When it became difficult to care for my menstruation and still go to school, I would say those words. When I became so angry that I wanted to retaliate, I would say those words. I knew it was okay to feel negatively sometimes, but those words reminded me that I could choose humility and gratitude even when it was difficult. I knew that my life could look healthy, happy, and holy because I could choose to think in this way and make decisions that led to positive outcomes."

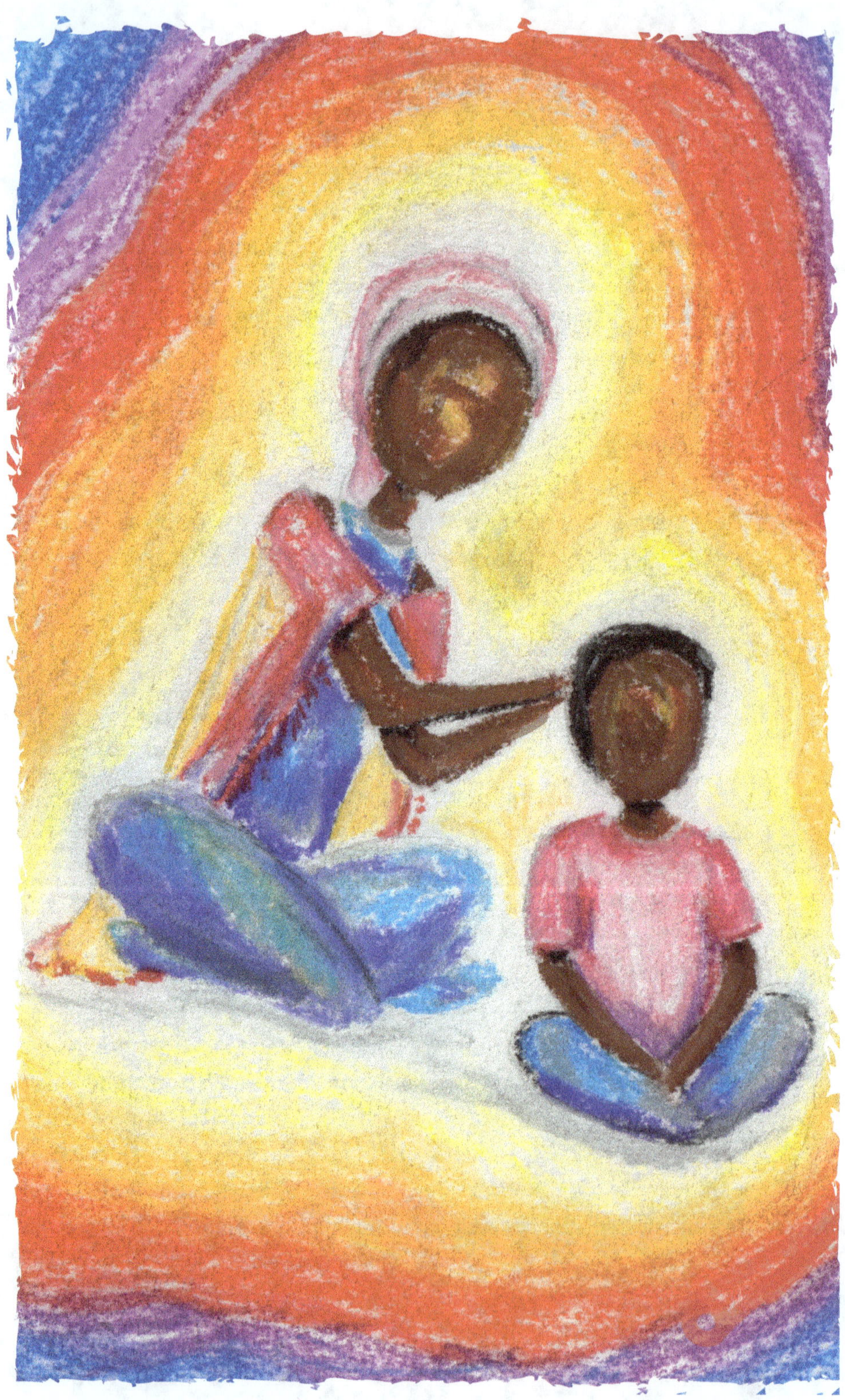

"Oh, Dr. Emma!" The girls hugged her tight. "We are so glad you made those choices and are here to help us." Dr. Emma returned their embrace with warmth and understanding, her heart swelling with pride at the impact of her life's work.

 Dr. Emma said, her eyes compassionate.

The girls settled in for this week's lesson.

"Yes! Thank you, Dr. Emma." The girls glanced at one another, chiming in unison with voices filled with newfound purpose and determination.

Listening intently, Farida spoke up, her voice trembling slightly. "Dr. Emma, I underwent FGM, and it has affected me deeply. How can I heal from this experience?"

Dr. Emma's expression softened with compassion.

Nyah, who had been quiet until now, finally spoke up, though her voice wavered with fear. "Dr. Emma, I am scared because my family wants to marry me off early. I do not want this. But, it is not my decision to make!"

Dr. Emma's reassuring smile comforted her.

The girls felt a sense of relief and empowerment, knowing they could trust Dr. Emma with their questions and concerns.

Pendo, Maryam, Farida and Nyah felt a new sense of purpose. As the sun set each day as they fetched water for their families, they discussed Dr. Emma's teachings and the difference this knowledge has made in their own lives. "Imagine, Maryam, if we could share Dr. Emma's wisdom with our friends, aunties, and mothers! Think of the difference it could make in our community if every woman understood her body!"

In Ubora village, despite the rich weaving of customs and culture, many things were not spoken of. Menstruation, the transition into womanhood, and having sex were a few of those things. Dr. Emma seemed to speak freely of these natural processes that were awkward for others to speak of. They were grateful to have her available to answer their questions and teach them things they had not thought to ask.

Pendo had noticed physical changes in her own body as she reached adolescence. Village women joked about what was occurring and used vague terms and half-truths. Pendo's mother and the other elderly ladies would quickly avert their gaze and speak quietly if she asked about it.

One afternoon, as Pendo and Maryam were fetching water along the dusty road, they discussed their growing understanding of women's health and the challenges their friends Farida and Nyah faced.

Pendo asked, "Maryam, do you ever wonder about... about when we become older? Why do we have to bleed? How do we become mothers? How can we prevent having more children than we care for? Do you think Farida knows how brave she is? To come here, despite her family's will?"

Pendo sighed. "And Nyah too. She's always so worried about being forced into marriage. How can we help her?"

"We need to encourage more girls and women to come to Dr. Emma's clinics. Understanding our bodies, our cycles, the choices we have is something we all need to know! And, if we discuss the dangers of FGM and early marriages, maybe they can change this tradition, just like Dr. Emma's mother did for her."

Pendo nodded. "Yes! We can talk to our aunties, mothers, and friends. Tell them about what we are learning from Dr. Emma. It could make a huge difference."

Waving her fingers in front of Maryam's face, Pendo leaned closer. "Why don't our parents or schools teach about it? Why the secrecy?"

Maryam exhaled, looking away. "Because of the old ways. I think most people do not understand the workings of women's bodies."

Maryam comforted Pendo. "You're right. What we do not understand about our bodies can hurt us. I have learned so much from Dr. Emma already. How can we care for something we know nothing about?"

Pendo nodded slowly, her gaze resolute. "I want to know how this part of life works. Dr. Emma has opened my curiosity and I want to keep learning. I feel there is so much more to know."

Maryam grinned, admiring her friend's determination. She raised her voice triumphantly. "Yes, Pendo, that is the spirit. Knowledge is power!" They chuckled as they kicked dust up along the path.

The next day as they joined Dr. Emma under the acacia tree, the girls eagerly shared their thoughts. "We were talking about how to encourage more women to come to your clinics. How can we help them understand?"

Dr. Emma smiled gently. "I can sense your passion for knowledge beyond tradition. There has been too much silence around your concerns for far too long."

Thrilled and excited, the girls exchanged glances, finding reassurance in Dr. Emma's words. "Then let's embark on a journey of science and wisdom together to dispel myths and break down taboos. Gather your trusted friends and family members and we will discuss and learn together."

Before Dr. Emma's next visit, Pendo, Maryam, Farida, and Nyah diligently gathered cousins, aunties, and even Pendo's grandmother. Some came hesitantly, afraid of exposing their ignorance, some refused, some were too busy with chores, while others eagerly embraced the opportunity to learn.

Those who came were initially nervous, but Dr. Emma's calm demeanor and kind words settled them. As she spoke, her words poured over them, reassuring them of their bravery in being there.

They listened attentively as Dr. Emma taught. "Every stage of life has new choices, new thoughts, and even new cells that make up our bodies. Life is change as witnessed in our bodies." Dr. Emma carefully took Pendo's grandmother by the arm and led her to one end of the women. She then took the baby off the back of

Maryam's 9-year-old cousin and placed her on the ground at the other end. Dr. Emma then escorted the rest and put them into age order, including Pendo, Maryam, Nyah and Farida in the middle.

Dr. Emma motioned to the baby cousin, stating, "It is a good thing we all start our lives as little and cute people because we need to be taken care of, and have very few choices to make. To grow and develop properly, every baby needs good nutrition, care, protection, and lots of love and guidance."

Dr. Emma then motioned to the middle group of girls. "In later childhood our bodies go through adolescence or puberty, marking the transition into adulthood. This is a crucial time of physical and emotional development."

"It is the process of becoming sexually mature—the body, not the mind—"

"—You can say that again." The aunties chuckled.

Dr. Emma continued, "Puberty typically occurs in girls aged 10 to 14, and boys aged 12 to 16. But there is no race in life. Just as in nature, there are slower-blooming and faster-blooming plants, and they are all beautiful in their own way. Look at this large acacia tree we are standing under. It is mature and has seed pods growing from it. It is in its reproductive years, just like these women here." The women and girls nodded in recognition while others absorbed the information with newfound understanding. Dr. Emma's inclusive approach created a safe space where questions were welcomed, and knowledge was shared openly.

Dr. Emma motioned to the aunties who had young children. She then pointed to a small twig coming out of the ground. "These small twigs can be just like this huge tree, but they are in the seedling stage, establishing their roots and leaf system and still need protection and care to become this beautiful, strong tree we are standing beneath. In between these stages is this time of puberty. In girls, it begins with breast growth, underarm and pubic hair, widening of the hips, deepening of the voice, and the beginning of her menstrual cycle, which marks the beginning of over 400 menstrual cycles for most women between the ages 12 and 51."

Pendo's eyes widened at the large number.

Dr. Emma motioned to Pendo's grandmother. "Menopause is when a woman has not menstruated or had no period for over a year. These women are in their wisdom years and are much needed in our societies for their experience and teachings. And like this beautiful tree that can now give protection and shade for all to gather under and learn."

"And the changes keep coming no matter our age." The grandmother chuckled. "That is why we say the only constant in life is change."

Dr. Emma smiled. "It is healthiest to view life's changes as opportunities. The more we grow through change and challenge, the stronger and better suited we are to help others through their challenges."

Dr. Emma picked up the baby and placed her by the grandmother, then waved the others forward to close the line and form a circle. Making the timeline into a circle drove her point home. "We all need each other to grow through challenges, strengthen one another, and share wisdom all throughout our lives."

Grandma swayed and started a familiar song of blessing and encouragement for the girls. As that song ended, another began. The unity felt there was strengthening to all.

At the end of a song, Maryam said, "This reminds me of Dr. Emma's mother's favorite song. Dr. Emma, will you teach them?"

"Of course, let's put our hands in the middle of the circle," Dr. Emma said. "This is a mantra for all the various stages of life and throughout the challenging circumstances of that time."

The women, girls, and even the babies joined hands and repeated after Dr. Emma, "Healthy am I, happy am I, holy am I."

After taking a collective peaceful exhale, Dr. Emma asked the group to return for her next visit to delve into the magnificence, mystery, and power of the female body. As they dispersed, Pendo, Maryam, Farida, and Nyah felt a renewed sense of purpose. They knew there was much work to be done in their community, but with Dr. Emma's guidance and their determination, they felt empowered to make positive change.

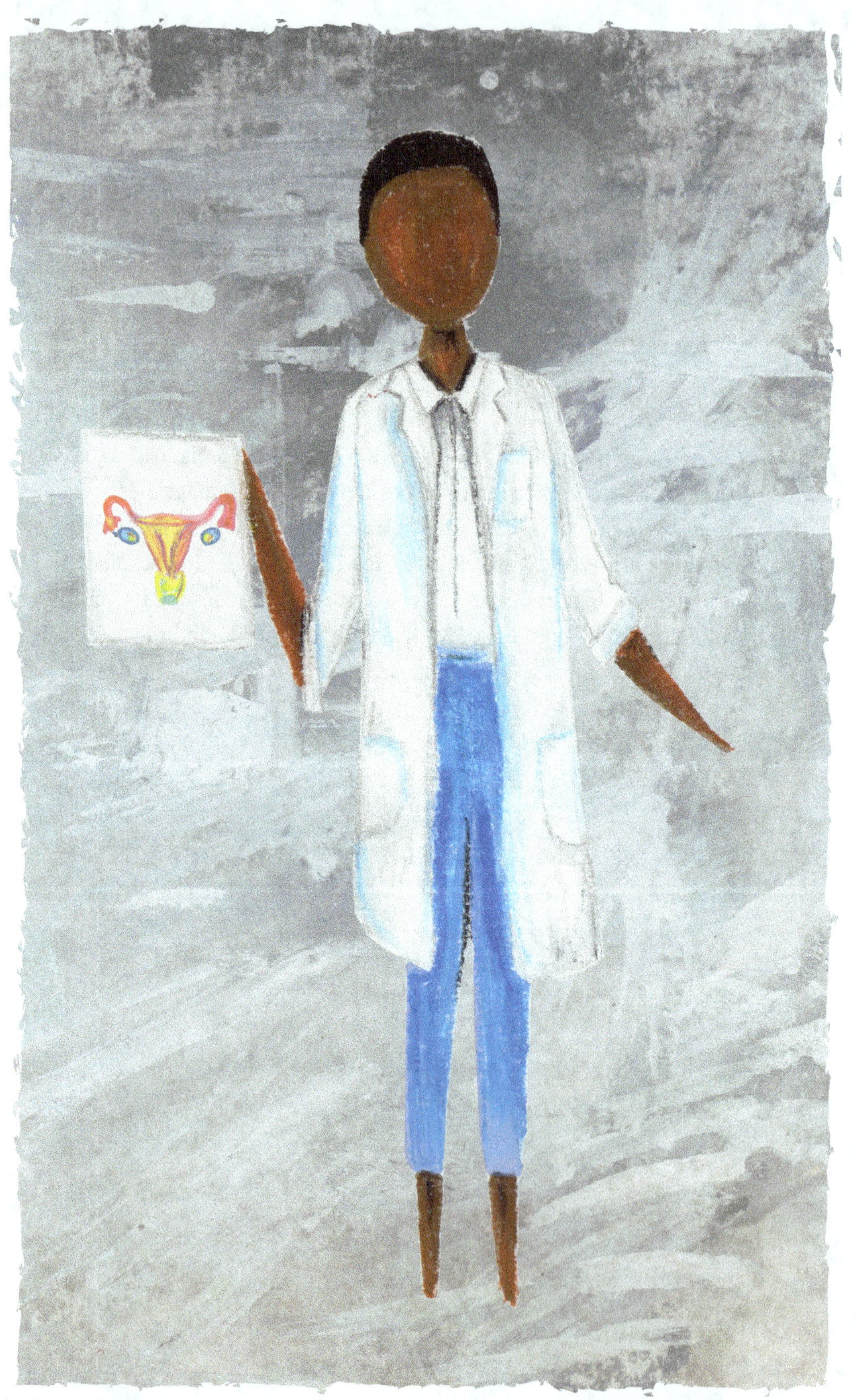

Chapter Three

$\mathcal{A}$ new trust had formed between the women of all ages. They faithfully continued to gather under the acacia tree each time Dr. Emma was scheduled to come to their village. As they assembled, they nervously giggled as they saw Dr. Emma holding a piece of paper in front of her hips. The women were eager to learn what those strange diagrams on the paper could mean.

"Our sexual organs are a great gift and need special care and concern. Caring for these sexual organs involves calling them by their proper and scientific names. By naming them, we will learn the amazing function they provide."

Dr. Emma then pointed to each part, naming and describing the organs. "The uterus is a hollow muscle about the size of your fist." She placed her fist over the cutout shape, representing the uterus. "This is the womb, where a fetus, or baby, develops after being conceived. The uterus goes through a cycle about every thirty days that builds up a soft lining. If a woman is not pregnant, the uterus sheds that lining and bleeds through her vaginal opening."

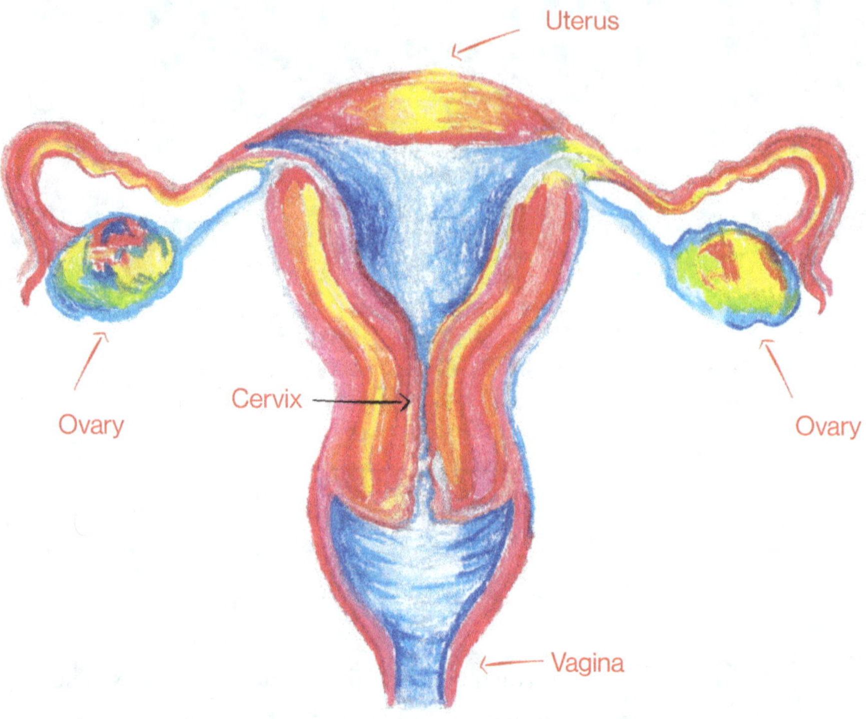

Dr. Emma clenched her fist in front of the picture.

"The blood comes from that muscle, the uterus?" asked Maryam.

"Is that why it hurts a bit sometimes, cramps up?" asked one of the aunties.

"That is right. Every month the lining in this hollow muscle gets thick and soft and sheds to start a new lining of blood for the next month. Menstruation is sometimes called a cycle or a period because it happens on a cycle for a period of time."

Dr. Emma put her thumb over the picture of the ovary. "These are called ovaries. Inside each ovary gland are millions of tiny cells called egg cells or ova. A tiny egg cell, no bigger than a pencil dot, bursts out of the ovary each month and begins the menstruation cycle. The ovaries, together with the uterus, also make chemicals called hormones that regulate the female reproductive system."

One of Pendo's cousins scrunched up her nose. "Why do we need to know all this science about our private parts?"

Grandmother spoke up. "I wish I had understood this when I started my cycle for the first time. I thought I was dying and felt ashamed and dirty. I never would leave the house and didn't know every woman experienced the same cycle. There were no doctors, no scientific explanation in my day. When I got married at a young age, I had no idea what part was what and no one to ask!"

"Let's discuss this next part, and I think your question will be answered." Dr. Emma presented another illustration depicting the exterior of the body, situated between the legs. "This tube connects the inside organs to the outside of the body. It is called a vagina, or a birth canal because it is a stretchy tube the baby comes through during birth. It is also the tube where the penis of a male is inserted during intercourse or sex. This tube also serves as a receptacle for tampons and menstrual cups to collect menstrual blood during your period. However, pads are positioned externally, resting in your underwear."

She pointed to the anatomy chart again. "There are three holes between your legs. The middle one is the vagina. The other holes are the urethra, where urine exits." She pointed to the upper hole. "And the anus." She pointed to the lower hole. "The urethra is the little tube where urine, or pee, comes out. The anus is where your poop comes out. The folds of skin protecting the urethra and vagina are called labia. The entire area is called the vulva."

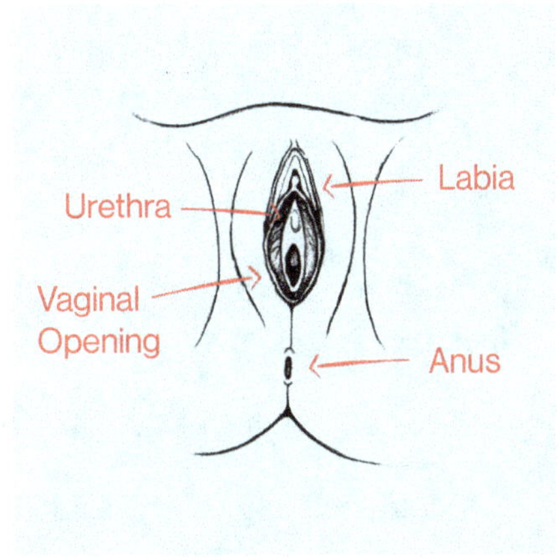

The girls' eyes glanced downward in embarrassment, and some aunties covered their mouths in surprise at the bluntness. Dr. Emma exhaled. "I know this can be embarrassing to discuss, but these private areas are very important." She pointed to an auntie. "Does this area of your body play a role in your health and the health of your family?"

The auntie sighed. "Yes. My children know when Mama is not feeling well. And my husband." She giggled. "Sometimes I get cramps so bad that I can't do chores, and I get infections quite regularly down there and even get fevers. How can I be healthy and not get infections?"

Dr. Emma held up the paper again and raised her voice. "These three holes are important to keep clean, which is not easy because they are so close to one another and can be quite delicate."

"Germs easily infect this genital region. Poop, or potty, from the anus, can carry many germs that can enter the bloodstream through the urethra." Dr. Emma pointed to the anus and then to the urethra. "Menstrual blood can also attract germs and cause infection." She pointed to the vaginal opening. "Sexual intercourse also introduces germs here through the abrasion and semen from the man. It is common for all women in all parts of the world to contract urinary tract infections especially where clean water is lacking. We can prevent many problems only if we know the correct information." She looked to the most embarrassed aunties. "You're all very brave for being here and learning."

Maryam interjected, "What is an infection, and what does it feel like?"

The aunties chuckled. "Urinating often. And it burns!"

"Foul-smelling urine," said another.

"Pain in the lower belly after urinating and pain in the lower abdomen and back," explained another.

"I had such a high fever once that my husband had to borrow a motorcycle to take me to the clinic," added the last auntie.

"Those sound like signs of an infection, all right. Fever, chills, and nausea are always signs that something is not right," Dr. Emma said. "Do you want to know how to prevent them?"

"YES!" they all shouted.

Dr. Emma held up seven fingers. "Drink lots of water to urinate often." She tucked her thumb. "Keep genitals clean, especially during menstruation and after pooping. If using toilet paper, wipe the urethra first and then your anus. Wear clean underwear every day of the month, and if using pads, change them daily. Wear soft pads and underwear that won't scratch or harm. Using items like rugs, dress fabric, mud, and leaves can harm the delicate urethra. Wear looser skirts, pants, and underwear to promote better airflow, and watch out for chemicals in cheap pads —they could cause irritation. If sexually active, make sure to wash well and urinate after sex, and never have sex with a partner who has a sexually transmitted disease."

"Cleanliness and care are essential," Dr. Emma said. "Just as we take care of our homes and fields, we must care for our bodies with diligence."

Dr. Emma took out a beautiful glass carafe of water and glasses. She carefully poured each of them a glass and proposed a toast. "Repeat after me," Dr. Emma said, "Healthy am I, happy am I, holy am I." The women eagerly joined in and downed their fresh, clean water.

With renewed resolve, the women gathered their belongings and bid farewell to Dr. Emma. Under the acacia tree Dr. Emma waved goodbye. "Next time, we will discuss the miraculous details of your cycle." Many walked home arm in arm, vowing to support each other through their challenges of womanhood, empowered with the knowledge of their beautiful anatomy. They were determined to spread awareness, support each other, and protect future generations.

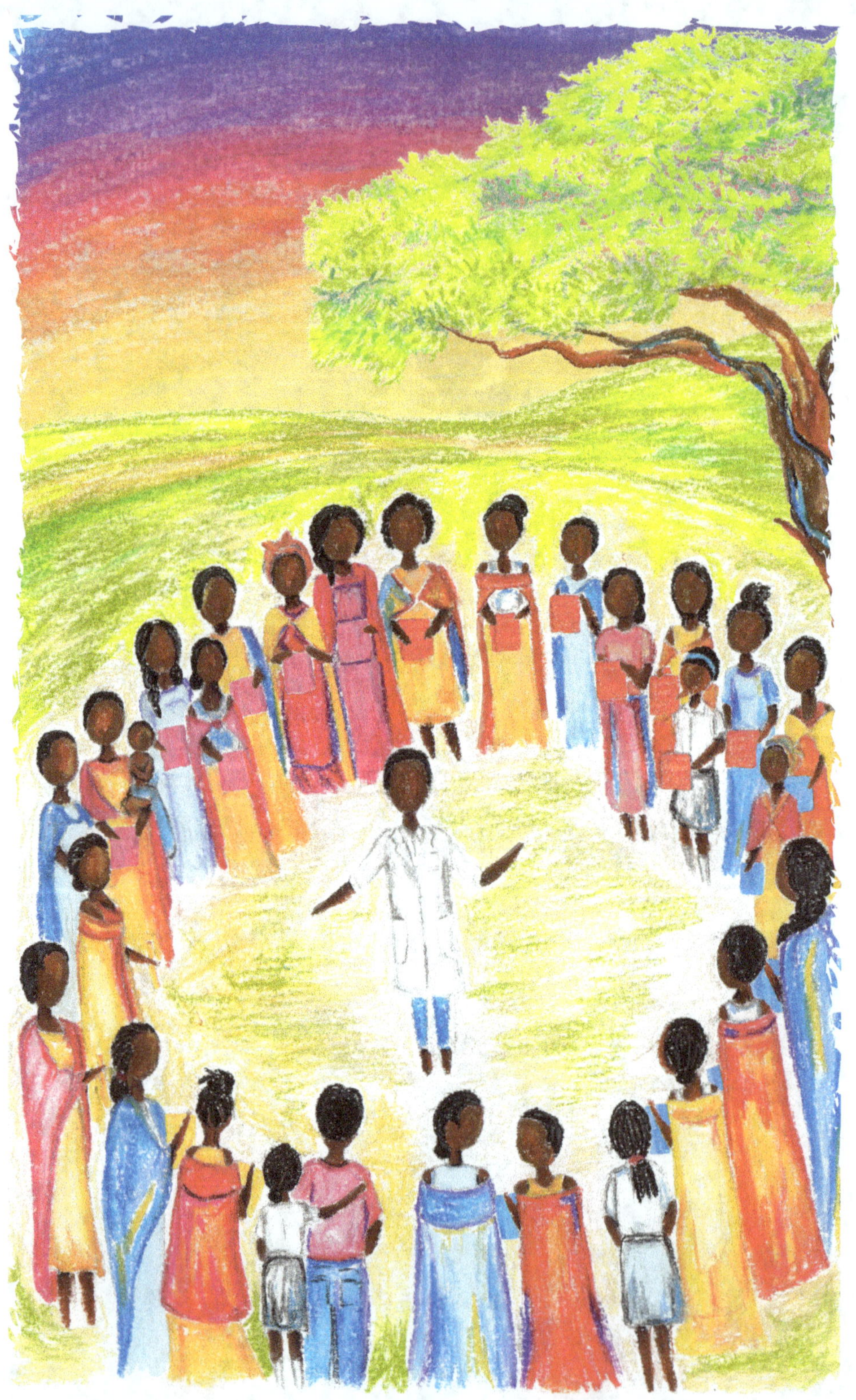

Chapter Four

____

The next time the women gathered under the sprawling acacia tree behind the clinic, they felt less embarrassed and ignorant. They were empowered to ask questions. A few more new friends, cousins, and curious acquaintances have heard of the important lessons happening behind the clinic.

"Dr. Emma, tell us more of your great facts," Maryam's grandmother said. "Why does our uterus need to bleed every month? We have many misunderstandings and wonder why it is considered taboo."

"And dirty and shameful," Pendo's cousin said.

Dr. Emma nodded. "That is why education and awareness matter. The boys' teasing of period accidents shows how these beliefs persist. The teasing has shaped our views for decades. It can be difficult to bleed every month, but it doesn't have to be."

Pendo went from curious to determined. "But we can change that, right? With knowledge and understanding?"

Hope shone through Dr. Emma's grin. "Yes, darling. The clinic I am creating will educate our town, not only heal sickness. We can break taboos when we learn science and recognize that there is nothing to fear. We can also easily access products to help us care for our periods hygienically and healthfully."

Maryam said, "We can feel healthy, happy, and holy even when we bleed?"

Dr. Emma nodded, beaming. "Indeed. It begins with discussions like this. We're pushing conventions and creating solutions. First, let us talk about *why* we menstruate and *how* to best care for ourselves."

Dr. Emma arranged the group in a circle. "The menstrual cycle is all about the state of the uterus." She handed seven women a piece of red paper. "These women represent the days of bleeding of the uterus." She held up a drawing of a uterus. "Remember this?"

"Yes," they all said.

"Where is the egg cell in this picture?"

"Isn't it so tiny we can't see it?" Maryam asked.

Dr. Emma nodded. "That is right, but it is there even though we can't see it. The week of bleeding, it is cleaned out of the uterus with all the blood and tissue of the inside of the uterus. Why do we care about that tiny egg cell anyway?"

Maryam's mother spoke up, "Because it is what can develop into a baby."

"That is right. An egg cell is released from the ovary every month. If it is fertilized, it will develop and grow inside the uterus for about 40 weeks. A woman knows she is not pregnant when this lining is shed. This is called your period—the period of time when you bleed. The blood slowly comes out through the vagina for about 3-7 days for most women."

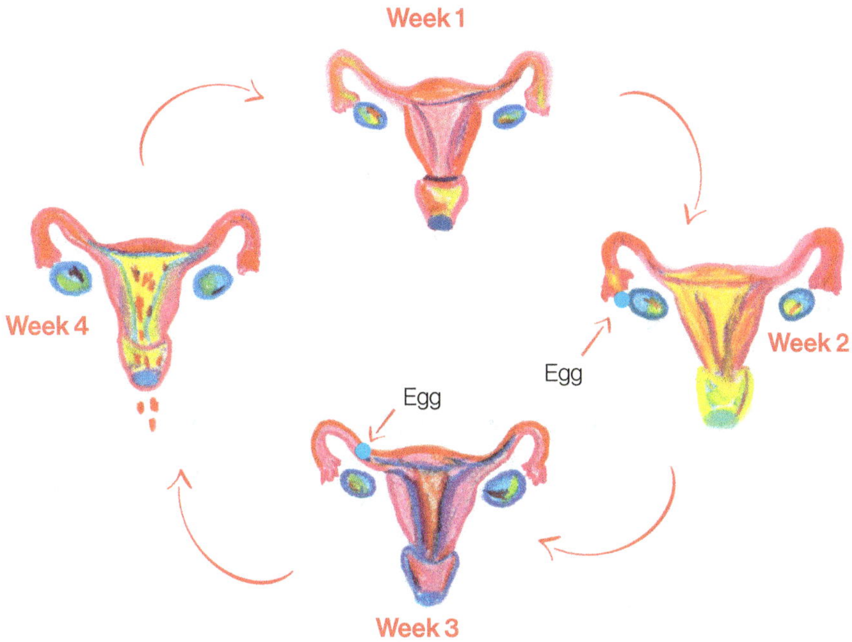

Next, Dr. Emma gave seven more women blue pieces of paper. She held up the diagram in front of her abdomen and explained. "The week after your period, a new egg cell develops in the ovary. The lining of the uterus will slowly thicken to allow the egg to be fertilized and implanted in later weeks. But, this week, it is like a thin blanket with no egg cells."

Dr. Emma handed out seven pieces of yellow paper. "These seven women represent the days of possible fertilization. The ovary releases an egg cell, and it travels down to the uterus. The uterus lining is thicker, and if a male's sperm meets the ovum during this week, a new human life can begin to implant in the uterus."

Dr. Emma handed out seven pieces of pink paper. Around the circle, twenty-eight women held a colored paper that represented the different weeks of the cycle—yellow, blue, pink, and red. "During this week, the egg cell travels to the uterus, and the lining of the uterus is its thickest and getting ready to shed. When your egg cell does not meet a man's sperm cell, the thick lining of your uterus is not needed because there is no baby to grow and nourish. Because the uterus is made of muscle, it can contract or cramp to release the unneeded tissue. It is preparing for the next week of period."

The women in the circle groaned. Dr. Emma laughed as she pulled one of the women into the middle. "Let's imagine that she is experiencing cramps today. She is miserable. What can be done to help her?"

"She can heat a warm towel and place it on her abdomen," one of the aunties said. "When I drink tea or a lot of water and move around, it helps, too. And you have a good medicine for pain at the clinic."

Dr. Emma nodded. "Yes, ibuprofen helps with cramps. We also tell her to breathe deeply and be gentle with herself. And what motto might help her?"

"Healthy Am I, happy am I, holy am I," they said in unison and laughed.

"But, Dr. Emma, how do we find happiness amidst the discomfort of cramps, accidental bleeding on our clothes, bad moods?" whined one of the aunties.

"That is a good question. Let's all sit and discuss what *happy am I* really means." As the women sat, Dr. Emma said, "I try to remember that I am only as happy as my thoughts. Who is in control of your thoughts?"

"I am. Most of the time…" Maryam chuckled. "Sometimes other people do not allow me to be happy, or when I am in pain or something embarrassing has happened."

Dr. Emma pulled Maryam to her in comfort. "Happy doesn't mean just pretending or pushing all negative emotions down only later to burst forth. Happy doesn't mean we feel happy only when everything is perfect in our situation."

"Because it never will be," Maryam's grandmother said.

"Many times, *happy am I* means *hopeful am I*." Dr. Emma said, with her hands on Maryam's shoulders. "We can have hope in any situation which will eventually lead to happiness. Let's put Maryam in a situation that is anything but happy and think of how she can turn negative or unhappy thoughts into more positive or hopeful thoughts."

Pendo said, "What if Maryam had a period accident at school? What if she wasn't prepared and got blood all over her school uniform?"

Maryam said, "Well, I wouldn't be thinking very happy thoughts. In fact, it can be so embarrassing that I wouldn't want to return to school."

Dr. Emma turned to the group. "What other thoughts would be natural to think?"

"I am disgusting."

"I am stupid and too poor to have the right supplies."

"I never want to come to school again."

"I should just stay home for the week of my period and not risk such things."

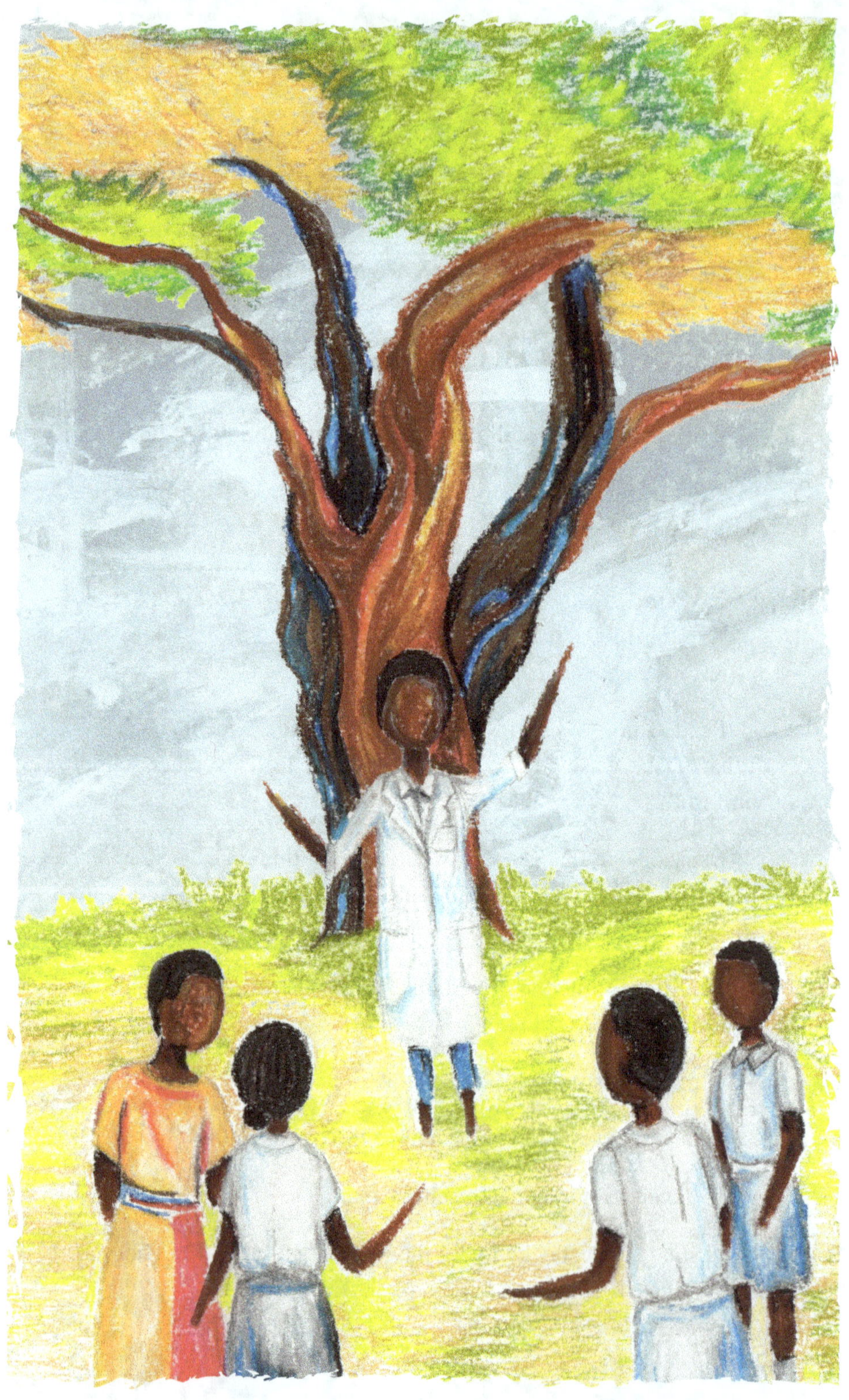

"This truly is a curse for women."

"Women are dirty and inferior."

Dr. Emma let the power and emotion of their feelings settle like the heavy heat beyond the shade of the acadia tree before speaking again. "Right. Not hopeful or happy. What will be the results of those thoughts?"

"The shame we've felt for too long," one auntie hung her head.

Dr. Emma leaned forward and gently lifted the auntie's head. "Do you believe that if that happened to Maryam, she should feel shame and embarrassment?"

"No, but what is happy or hopeful about that situation, Dr. Emma?"

Dr. Emma turned to the group. "What can we think when shameful thoughts come our way?"

The women looked puzzled until some ideas started being voiced. "Oh no, I have had an accident. Accidents happen."

"She can be humble and ask a friend for assistance."

"I can learn from this mistake, calendar my period, and bring supplies with me most of the week I am expecting my period."

"At least I am not pregnant!" the auntie said, laughing.

The mood lightened and Dr. Emma said, "Feelings stem from our thoughts. I feel hopeful when I hear thoughts that have a sense of humor or help me learn wisdom or thoughts that I am capable of even when humbled."

Maryam smiled. "I feel much better now, thank you. It seems that by thinking those hopeful thoughts I will be more likely to learn from not being prepared. I can choose to keep going to school instead of hiding my head in shame and never going back."

Hope filled the air.

Farida raised her hand. "Dr. Emma, can we talk about the costs of menstrual supplies? Many of us cannot afford to buy pads every month."

"Yes!" Dr. Emma said. "That is a crucial part of our discussion. Period poverty is when a woman cannot afford or acquire the means for menstrual supplies. It keeps women from attending school or working or even from caring for themselves and their families."

Dr. Emma's heart held the memories of her childhood village. She had grown up alongside her best friend, Emily, their dreams intertwined like vines in the forest. However, their aspirations were thwarted by the relentless force of period poverty and the weight of tradition.

"In my village," Dr. Emma began, her eyes distant, "there was a time when menstrual supplies were as scarce as rain in a drought. We wore the same lightweight, see-through uniforms as you do. But there was something even more challenging than the lack of pads—the head teacher, a stern man, believed girls should not attend school during their periods."

Dr. Emma's gaze lingered on the young faces before her. "Emily, my dearest friend, faced the brunt of this unjust belief. She would stay home during her period week, month after month, her education slipping away like grains of sand through her fingers."

As Dr. Emma spoke, the fire in her eyes intensified, recalling Emily's lack of choices. "Desperation drove her into the arms of a Sugar Daddy, a man who promised to fund her education in

But dreams can be shattered in the harsh light of reality. Dr. Emma's voice trembled with emotion as she shared the painful truth. "Emily became pregnant and was cast out of her home, left to raise her baby alone. The very dreams she had sacrificed everything for crumbled before her."

Pendo and Maryam exchanged solemn glances, understanding the gravity of Dr. Emma's words. The story served as a poignant reminder of the vicious cycle countless girls faced.

Dr. Emma's eyes turned sad. "Emily and I remained friends." Her voice carried the weight of shared determination. "We vowed that no other girl should endure what she went through. We decided to change the narrative, to break the trap that forces girls to sell their bodies for necessary items."

It was Maryam's turn to put a comforting hand on Dr. Emma's shoulder. "Thank you for helping us."

"When a woman, whether young or older, views herself as someone worthy of happiness, health, and holiness, she will make the best decision at that particular moment in her menstrual cycle. Next time, I will bring options for women to choose from, each with pros and cons so we can discuss ways to combat period poverty and make these options available."

The group formed a circle, their voices joining in harmony and, this time, with more conviction than ever. **"Healthy are we, happy--"**

"And hopeful!"

"--are we, holy are we."

Chapter Five

The following week a table sat beside the tree with items and a chart. Dr. Emma greeted the women and was pleased to see new faces.

"So happy to see all of you today. Some of these menstrual options are modern, and some of are traditional. Each woman gets to choose the best option for her at different times of her life. Here are six options. They each have positive and negative aspects. Let's go through them so you are well informed about your best choice."

Dr. Emma picked up the disposable pad. "What are the advantages of this most typical type of menstrual product?"

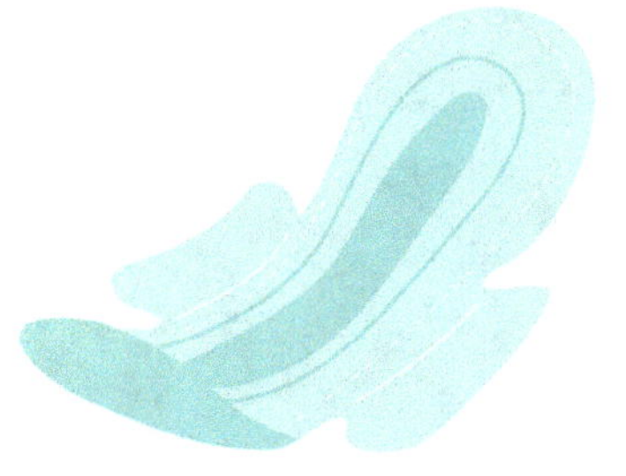

"Easy to use."

"Few health risks."

"Easily accessible."

"No need to wash or dry; just throw away or burn."

Dr. Emma added, "There are disadvantages as well. They can be expensive, have a high environmental impact as some pads have plastics and adhesives to dispose of, can cause a foul odor or infection. And, if not changed often enough, and can cause leakage and odor and staining of clothing. There are, however, pads that are made from natural materials that are better for the environment as they decompose quickly. Any material that comes in contact with this delicate and highly vulnerable area of the body, needs to be free from toxins, dyes, chemicals, and bleach."

"And not be scratchy or cause a rash," one auntie said.

Pendo's younger cousin picked up a tampon. "What is this thing? Do I want to know?" She covered her eyes.

Auntie said, "That is called a tampon. We do not have such things available around here. This goes into the vagina to soak up the blood, but our traditions say it is not wise to insert, especially for young girls. Are these safe, Dr. Emma?"

Dr. Emma nodded. "It is not the best choice for those who do not want to insert anything into the body. However, the best thing about tampons is the ease of use during sports, or swimming. They are also easy to dispose of. However, the worrisome part is that they must be changed every few hours as they can harbor bacteria and cause internal infections. It is also very important to use non-toxic tampons. The vaginal tissues are very delicate and can absorb toxins easily from bleaches or chemicals used in some brands of tampons."

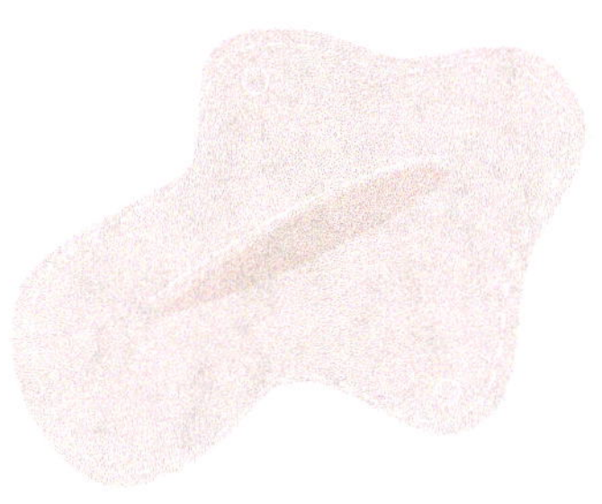

Grandmother picked up a reusable cloth pad. "These can be very nice. My friend was taught to make these, and they can last many years if properly washed and dried. Unfortunately, they can be expensive to make although they will be much less expensive than disposable pads over time. My niece used them and said the washing is not difficult. Sometimes when the sun is not as hot that day, the drying takes longer than she is able to wait. My daughter said she is embarrassed for her family to see her pads drying. I suppose that is a con for her."

Dr. Emma said, "Right, reusable cloth pads have many positive aspects and some negative. Depending on the amount of your flow and how often one needs to change them, they can be handy and gentle for both the user and the environment."

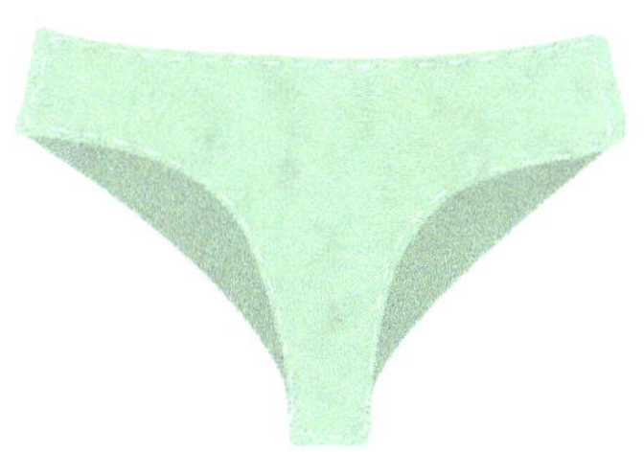

Nyah was examining a pair of underwear that was extra padded in the middle and another pair with less padding. "These are called period panties," she said, holding up the padded pair. The girls were awed at the quality.

Dr. Emma said, "These can be expensive, but also an investment as they will absorb blood and prevent leakage through a woman's clothes and useful for all women who suffer urine leaks. They are especially nice to sleep in and can be worn with a pad, tampon, or cup for extra assurance. And, like reusable pads, they need to be appropriately soaked, washed, and dried." She held up the less padded pair. "These are good quality underwear that are non-toxic and breathable. These are not expensive but are a good fabric that will allow breathability in the crotch area. One would want to wear pads, tampons, or a cup with these, or these can be worn anytime of the month and provide good coverage yet have no risk of harboring bacterial or fungal growth from trapped moisture. Remember it is normal to have discharge, or a mucus-like discharge from the vagina anytime of the month. That is why it is important to wear clean underwear every day. There is a sense of dignity that comes with good underclothing, and I would hope every girl and every woman has a few pairs of good quality underwear."

Maryam picked up a small, soft, rubberish cup. "This is a reusable cup. It is worn inside and is very hygienic as it doesn't absorb blood. It collects the blood and can be emptied out as needed. The nice thing about a cup is how long a woman may keep it in and easily wash it for the next period."

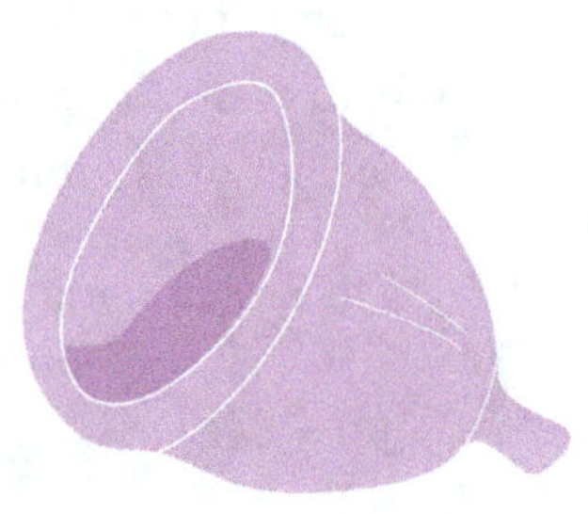

"Does it hurt to insert?" asked one of the cousins.

"Not at all," Dr. Emma answered. "This is the product I use monthly. I just fold it in half and insert it. I use my fingers to safely make sure it expands against the cervix to collect the blood like a cup."

Dr. Emma noticed the horrified look on the young girls' faces. "It can be scary and takes time and maturity to learn. It is the most hygienic, least expensive, and easy-to-use menstruation product. This is why we are discussing many choices. I am comfortable with my anatomy and do not have religious concerns about inserting anything in the vagina. When I use it with period underwear or small pad I never worry about leaking. I can work and travel between villages all day. It takes practice to insert and take out and is best done where water is available to wash hands before and after. It is nice to wash the vulva area as well every time. Some girls in schools carry a small cup of water into the toilet area with them to wash up. It can be a great option with long-lasting benefits. It can last for years if washed with very hot water every month, making it affordable and eco-friendly."

Dr. Emma stood in front of the table of products. "These each have pros and cons. It is up to each woman and young woman to decide how she cares for her menstruation. What is best for you, the environment, and what you can afford, and access will be different for each of you and at other times of your life. And can also change from month to month, which is okay, too. Just remember that it needs to support your healthy, happy, and holy self."

The group nodded in agreement.

Grandma looked at each girl. "Dear girls, let me know how I can support you so you always feel prepared. I want you to have the ability to care for this part of your body. My friends and I can sew reusable pads for you, at the very least. There are always options for you. Please come talk to me."

Dr. Emma gave Grandma's arm a nudge. "Thank you, Grandma. That kind of support and wisdom will allow the girls to keep going healthy and strong during all the days of the month. Next time we gather, we will discuss how to predict when your period is coming, to assure you will be prepared to meet the day… every day. In our discussion, we can also address the very needful topic of how to prevent or enable pregnancy."

Faridah raised her hand shyly. "Dr. Emma, I have a question. What if we do not have access to clean water all the time? How do we keep everything clean?"

Dr. Emma smiled warmly. "That is a very important question. If clean water is not always available, you can carry a small container of clean water with you, especially when you know you will need to change or clean your menstrual products. It is also helpful to have a small towel or cloth to dry your hands. Using natural, unscented wet wipes can also be an option in a pinch but remember to dispose of them properly. The key is to do the best you can with what you have and make sure to clean your hands and menstrual products thoroughly whenever possible."

Nyah said, "I think I want to try making the reusable pads. They seem like a good balance between cost and being kind to the environment."

Dr. Emma nodded approvingly. "That is a wonderful idea. And remember, you have the support of Grandma and her friends to help you learn how to make and care for them."

The women put their hands in a circle. **"Healthy am I, happy am I, holy am I."**

"Every day of the month," Dr. Emma added wholeheartedly.

Disposable Pad

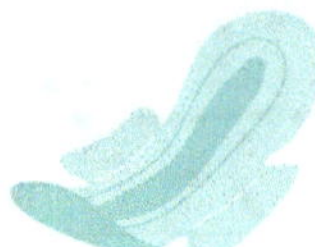

Pros	Cons
• Easy to use • Few health risks • Used only externally • Easy to find in stores globally • When you're done, you throw them away	• Doesn't hold much menstrual flow • Can be expensive • Has a high environmental impact • Can cause bad odor • Contain bleaches, plastics, • adhesives and chemicals

Tampon

Pros	Cons
• Less odor during use • Can be used while swimming/ sports • Tampons are not as noticeable as wearing pads • Can hold more flow than pads	• Must be changed every few hours • Higher risk of vaginal infections • Can leak • Not acceptable in some cultures or religions • Can increase menstrual cramps.

Reusable Cloth Pads

Pros	Cons
• Reusable • Will not chafe or irritate skin • Thinner than disposable pads • May last up to five years • No environmental impact	• Some trial and error in figuring out how to use them properly • Must be washed after each use • Need to carry a bag to store your used pads when they are full • There's a stigma surrounding cloth pads for some people • It can be expensive to start

Period Underwear

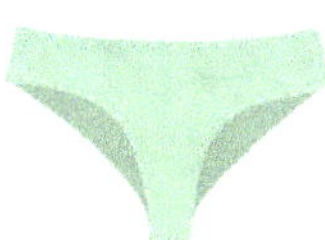

Pros
- Easy to use
- Used externally, so it is accepted by religions and cultures
- No environmental impact

Cons
- Expensive initial investment
- Must be purchased online or made Must be soaked, washed, and dried.
- Can cause odor overtime.

Menstrual Cup

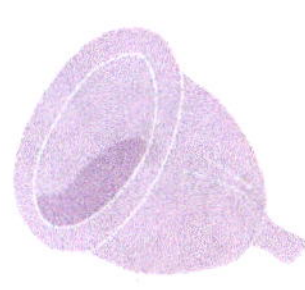

How to Insert: Fold it so it looks like a tampon, aim it toward the back of the vagina and give a little push. It should draw itself up. When inserted properly, you shouldn't feel its presence at all.

Pros
- No costs after initial investment
- No environmental impact
- No embarrassing odor
- Hygienic with little to no infection risk
- More time between changes. You can go up to 12 hours, depending on flow, with a menstrual cup before emptying
- Easy to use.

Cons
- Can be difficult to insert for young girls and those who've never had intercourse.
- It is possible to have fit problems. Sometimes individual anatomy can make proper use of the cup difficult.
- Removing the cup takes practice
- After each cycle the cup must be washed. It's best to have running water when emptying.
- Not acceptable in some cultures or religions.

Rags/ Toilet Paper

Pros
- Inexpensive and available

Cons
- They are a high infection risk and easily attract bacteria
- High risk of leaking
- Difficult to manage and keep in place
- Can trap odor
- Can be abrasive to genital
- may cause infection

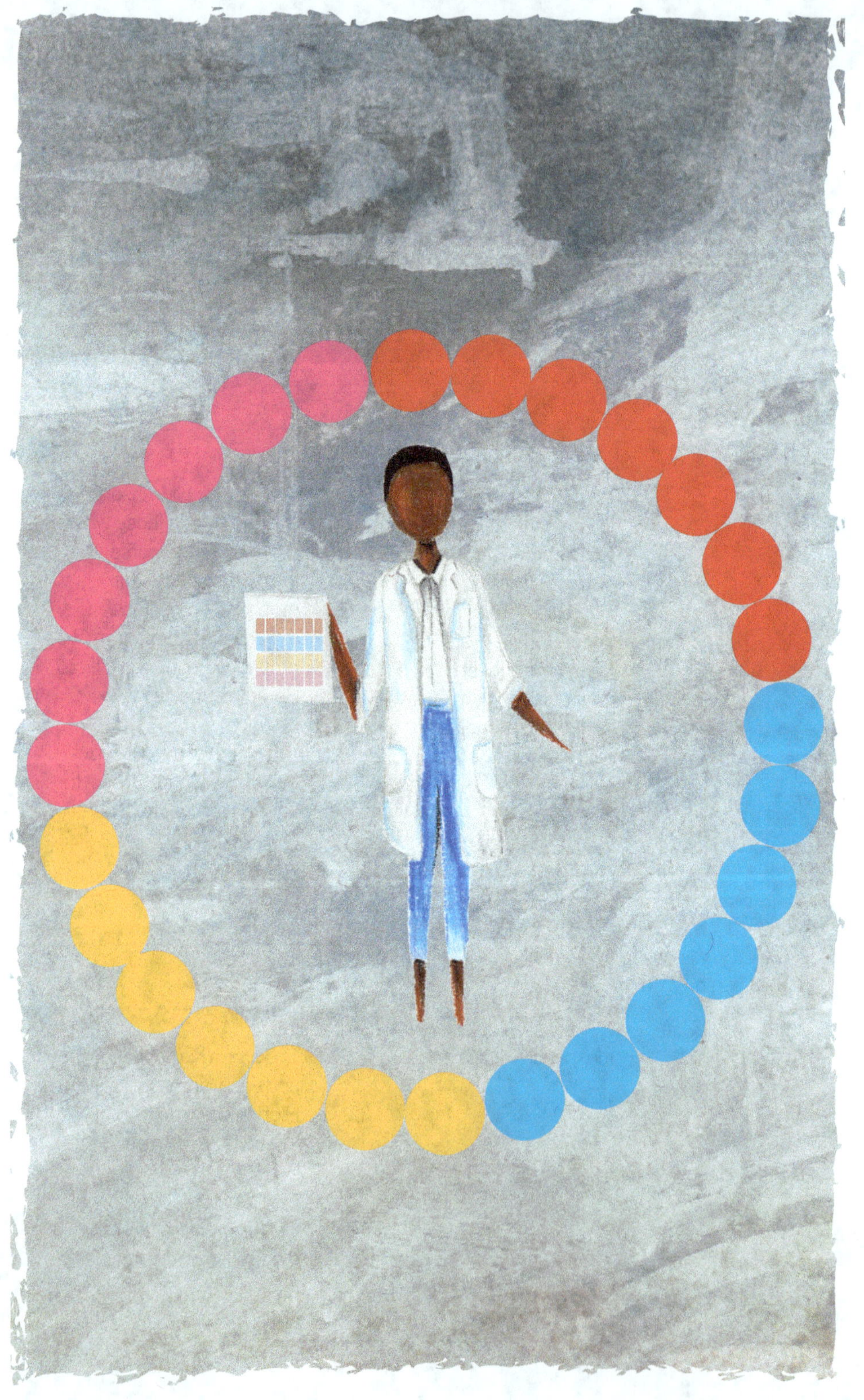

Chapter Six

---

*D*r. Emma began the new week's discussion with a warm smile. "Today, we are going to add to what we know about menstruation, a natural part of every woman's life, understanding this process and how to manage it with dignity."

The elder aunties had asked Dr. Emma if they could share their wisdom. One of them, Auntie Nia, said, "Thank you, Dr. Emma, for always reminding us that menstruation is a normal, healthy function of a woman's body. It signifies the potential to create life and should not be a source of shame or secrecy."

Dr. Emma nodded in agreement. "That is right, Auntie Nia. This knowledge helps us stay prepared and informed."

Pendo, Maryam, Farida, Nyah and the other girls listened intently as Dr. Emma explained the importance of maintaining a menstrual calendar. "Keeping a record of your menstrual cycle is valuable for multiple reasons," Dr. Emma said. "It helps you predict when your next period will arrive, allowing you to be prepared. It is also crucial for family planning, should you choose to use it."

"A girl should not be given power over a man to decide such things," a voice from the group bellowed.

The group turned to see who was talking. It was a new member of the group, a middle-aged woman Pendo recognized as a family friend. She and her mother spoke often. Her name is Fatima. She introduced herself boldly.

Dr. Emma acknowledged the opposing view. "Hello, Fatima. We want to hear your opinion, please go on."

Fatima stood up, her face stern. "In our tradition, men are the heads of households. They decide when to have children and how many to have. Giving women control over such matters disrupts the natural order and leads to disrespect and disobedience."

A murmur spread through the group. Some nodded in agreement, while others seemed troubled. Pendo felt a rush of shame flood her mind. It is this tradition particularly that hung over the heads of most girls. She stood speechless while her heart raced.

Thankfully, Dr. Emma maintained her calm. "I understand your concern, and it is important to respect our traditions. However, it is also crucial to understand that family planning is not about taking power away from men. It is about working together as partners to ensure the health and well-being of the family. When women can track their cycles, they can better communicate with their husbands about the best times to conceive or avoid pregnancy. It is a shared responsibility. When men and women work together in decision making, especially concerning family planning, it will surely end in a better result. Fatima, do you mind telling us how this has played out in your life?"

Fatima's face fell as she told of her many pregnancies that ended in miscarriage. She felt as though she was pregnant or nursing or both for decades. She recounted carrying a toddler on her back while nursing a newborn. Her milk would dry up quickly because she was unable to properly rest and feed herself and her children. Her voice rose in volume as she straightened her posture. "I always felt it was an honor to my husband to have many children. I do wonder if my body and my children's bodies would have been healthier to have more years between pregnancy and breastfeeding before getting pregnant again." Her eyes looked upward as she shrugged her shoulders. "I was only being obedient to my husband, and my husband does not know about my health like I do."

Dr. Emma looked Fatima in the eyes. "Fatima, you are quite right. It is tradition to be obedient to your husband. Do you feel though that it is honoring him to bring forth children you and he are unable to care for?"

Fatima looked away thoughtfully. "To tell you the truth I never felt there was another way. I was circumcised before I was given in marriage to my husband. My husband was wealthy and paid my parents a large dowry. I felt successful in a way, to my family to be able to provide for them security. It was then my duty to satisfy him and give him children, in return for the large dowry he had paid. He was fifteen years older than me and has since died. I, like many widows, must now work hard to provide for myself and my children. Dr. Emma, are you saying all this tradition is not good? Are you saying my husband and I did everything wrong?"

Dr. Emma took a deep breath. "You were not wrong, Fatima, you only did what you knew. This very question is why I am here. Learning facts can challenge these traditions that ultimately bring sorrow into our culture. There is another way, a healthier, happier, and holier way. A way that opens up possibilities and choices."

"What is circumcision? Why do people do this?" asked Nyah.

"Circumcision for females is also termed Female Genital Mutilation, or FGM, there are various forms of FGM, ranging from the partial or total removal of the clitoris to more extensive procedures that involve stitching the vaginal opening," Dr. Emma said. "It is not only a violation of their rights but also a significant health risk. FGM can cause chronic pain, infections, complications in childbirth, and even death. It is important to understand that FGM does not have any health benefits; it is rooted in cultural beliefs. These cultural beliefs plague our society and endanger the lives of millions of girls who live in East Africa, West, Central and North Africa, Yemen, Iraq, Indonesia and Malaysia. Sadly, the rates of FGM among us has only gone up in recent years. This mutilation needs to be challenged and changed. Only the women, especially those who've seen the negative consequences in their own lives, can change the culture or this practice."

Fatima said, "Many believe FGM is necessary for a girl to become a respectable woman. How can we change such deep-rooted beliefs?"

Dr. Emma nodded. "Changing such beliefs takes time and education. It involves having open conversations like this one, where we can discuss the facts and health risks associated with FGM. It is important to note that it is the women in most cases that refuse to stand up for the young girl in danger of enduring FGM. It is a betrayal at the very core for a girl to be harmed in this way by other women who know and understand its detrimental effects."

Pendo, feeling encouraged, spoke up. "What about early and forced marriages? How does that impact our health and rights?"

Dr. Emma looked around the circle, ensuring she had everyone's attention. "Early and forced marriages are significant issues that affect the health, education, and future of young girls. Marrying young often leads to early pregnancies, which carry higher risks of complications and sometimes death. It often means the end of a girl's education, limiting her opportunities for personal and economic development. Usually forced marriages are to older men which means that for most of the woman's life she will be a widow. It makes more sense to advocate for girls to complete their education and reach an age where they can make informed decisions about marriage and family planning. More choice means more life satisfaction and joy."

Nyah, with a serious expression, raised her hand again. "Dr. Emma, what can we do to protect young girls from forced marriages and FGM? It seems that no one will listen to our opinion."

Dr. Emma nodded. "That's a great question, Nyah. You asking those questions is helping this cause. You have the facts now, you can talk respectfully and truthfully and, most importantly, boldly about these practices to anyone. If you know anyone in danger of these practices you can help her find support or safety."

She continued talking to the group. "All of us can help empower girls with knowledge and self-confidence. This means providing them with education and vocational training so they can be self-reliant. Then, we must work with local leaders and policymakers to create and enforce laws that protect girls from being forced into marriage."

Auntie Nia added, "I intend to create a safe space where girls can speak out and seek help if they are being pressured into marriage. We need to support each other as a community."

Fatima folded her arms tighter, but there was a thoughtful look on her face. "I see your points, but I can't imagine as a young

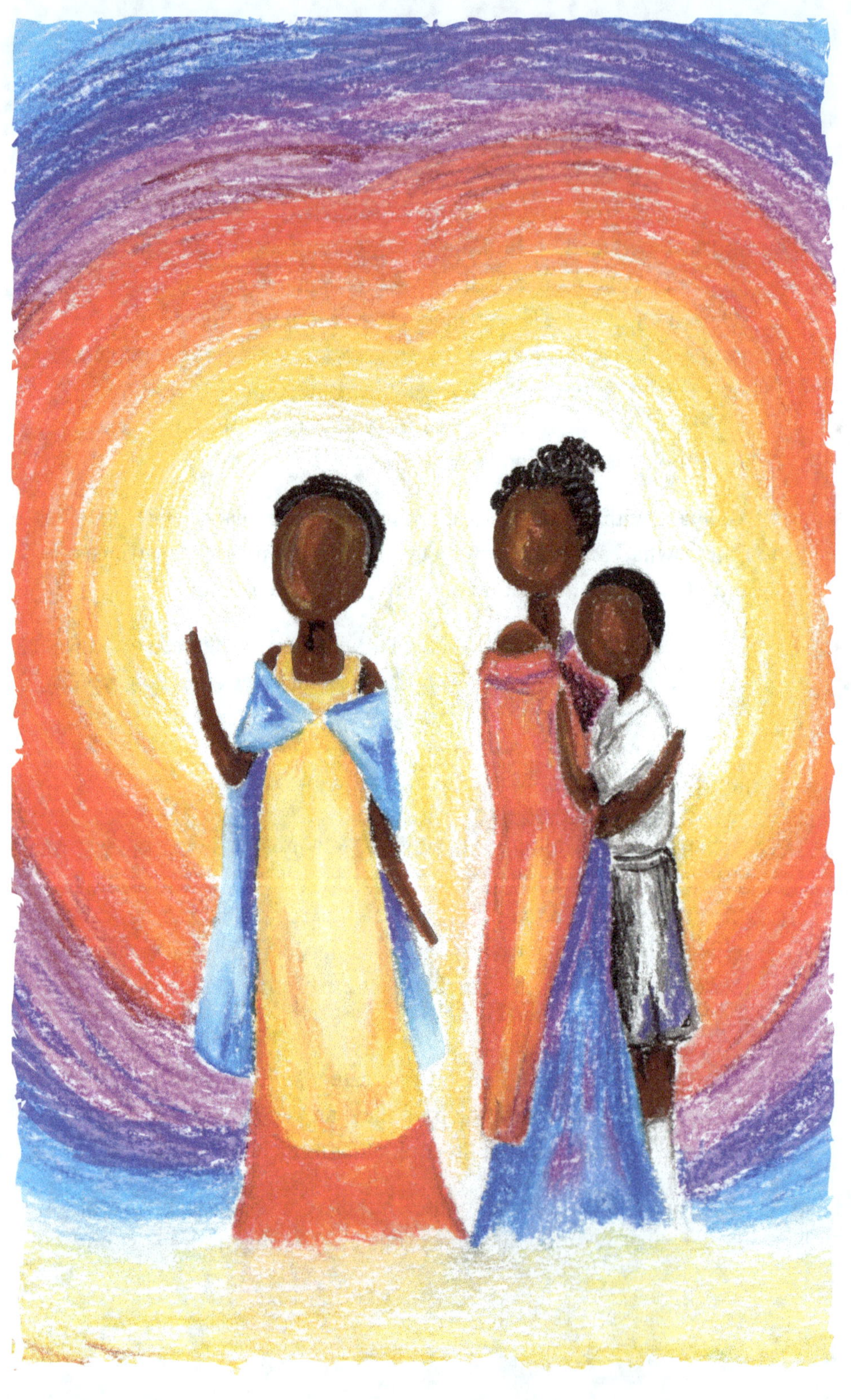

girl being able to say no to FGM and arranged marriage. It seems impossible to change traditions."

Dr. Emma smiled warmly. "You probably didn't know better as a young girl, did you?"

"Absolutely not." Fatima grimaced at the memory.

"It is not about abandoning our traditions, but about evolving them to protect and empower our women and girls. This discussion we've had today alone will save many, many girls from FGM because now that you know, you will not stand by and allow it happen to anyone you love. Am I right?"

The group nodded in agreement, feeling a sense of unity and purpose. Grandma stepped forward, her voice strong and reassuring. "Dear girls, all of us have the power to support each other. Let us use this knowledge to care for our bodies, our daughters, and our community. We are stronger together."

Grandma then jokingly asked Dr. Emma, "Let's say we actually did have a say on who to marry and when. How does a woman control when she gets pregnant?"

Dr. Emma reminded them of the circle they created and the yellow-colored fertile days. "It is most important to know that by choosing to have sexual intercourse, a woman chooses the possibility of becoming pregnant. However, she can mitigate the risk by knowing some key scientific facts about her cycle and the timing of when she has sex. Let's revisit our circle once more as a reminder."

As the circle formed, Dr. Emma passed out the colored papers. "Try and arrange yourselves into a cycle circle."

The women formed a circle with each week as a different paper color. Dr. Emma pointed to the yellow week. "Remember, these are the days the egg cell is available and viable to meet the male sperm cell through intercourse. If this happens, a new life begins to form."

One of the older girls spoke up. "What if we aren't ready to become a mother and also can't afford modern family planning methods like contraceptives or menstrual tracking apps?"

"It is essential to remember that there are traditional methods that can be cost-effective and accessible. Some women in our village have been using natural methods like calendar tracking and understanding their body's signals for generations. These traditional methods can be just as effective when used correctly. The key is to learn how to identify your fertile days and act accordingly, whether you are trying to conceive a baby or prevent pregnancy."

Maryam had a follow-up question. "Wait, what are contraceptives?"

Dr. Emma smiled at Maryam's curiosity. "Modern contraceptives are things such as birth control pills, injections, and intrauterine devices. They can be highly reliable in preventing pregnancy. However, it is important to consult a healthcare professional to determine which method suits you and to consider potential side effects. Contraception pills control the egg cell through hormones in the pill. It must be taken daily, costs, and has side effects."

Dr. Emma continued, "And remember, any family planning decision should be made after careful consideration and discussion with your partner. It is a choice that should be made together. If your partner is responsible and truly cares for you, he will have

There were some knowing chuckles from the older women.

"It is not easy to be responsible in the heat of the moment," Nia added.

"This all seems so serious," moaned Maryam.

Grandmother consoled them. "It is the most important decision and responsibility of your life. Your children and family are your richest treasure. You want to be ready, and able and have a supportive husband to help you love and raise your children."

"It seems as though women do not get the final say on these matters," Maryam said, looking down at her feet sadly.

Pendo, with a determined look in her eyes, approached the group. Her friend Grace had agreed to come and stood beside her. Pendo had made a promise to herself and to Grace that she would help her find support and guidance from Dr. Emma and the group.

Grace stood nervously beside Pendo. She had heard about Dr. Emma and the group's discussions and had finally found the courage to seek their assistance.

Pendo introduced Grace to Dr. Emma and the group. "This is Grace. She has been through a lot, and she needs our help. She's determined not to fall into the Sugar Daddy trap and wants to finish her education."

Grace, her eyes filled with fear and hope, looked at the group of women and girls. Dr. Emma, her voice gentle and reassuring, spoke to her.

The other girls in the group nodded in agreement, offering Grace their support and understanding. They could sense the determination in Grace's eyes and were ready to stand by her side as she worked to shape her future, free from the traps that had ensnared many girls in their village.

Grace, her voice still tinged with nervousness, began to speak. "I... I want to share something with all of you." She took a deep breath, steadying herself, and continued. "I have been struggling with a difficult decision." Tears welled up in Grace's eyes as she recounted her harrowing experience. "A boda-boda taxi driver drove me to a secluded spot and took advantage of me. He raped me. It felt like the world was closing in on me. I kept replaying the situation in my mind, and wondered how I could've prevented that. Could I have done something differently? I began to see myself as worthless…used goods. I just do not feel like the girl I once was, the girl who had a bright future."

The group listened in rapt silence, empathizing with Grace's difficult situation. It was common for men to see young girls as just something to consume and disrespect.

"I thought about compromising my education to avoid any shame and humiliation, but I do not want that anymore. I want to finish my education and I want to break free from the trap of low expectations for women. I want to have a family in the future, just not right now. I want a healthy family with a husband who respects me."

Dr. Emma, her gaze full of compassion, spoke to Grace.

Pendo, who had stood by Grace's side throughout, added, "You're not alone in this journey, Grace. We are here to support you every step of the way."

As Grace stood before the group, her trembling slowly subsided, replaced by a glimmer of hope. The support and understanding she received from Pendo, Dr. Emma, and the other girls gave her a renewed sense of determination.

The other girls in the group nodded in agreement, offering Grace their unwavering support. This was a pivotal moment in Grace's life. She realized that she had allies who would help her protect her future without compromising her integrity.

"My goal is to be Happy, healthy, and holy–even when others do not treat me as such." Grace straightened her shoulders. Fatima put her arm around Grace as if to show she had been there.

"Healthy am I, happy am I, holy am I." The group closed this week's meeting feeling more united than ever before.

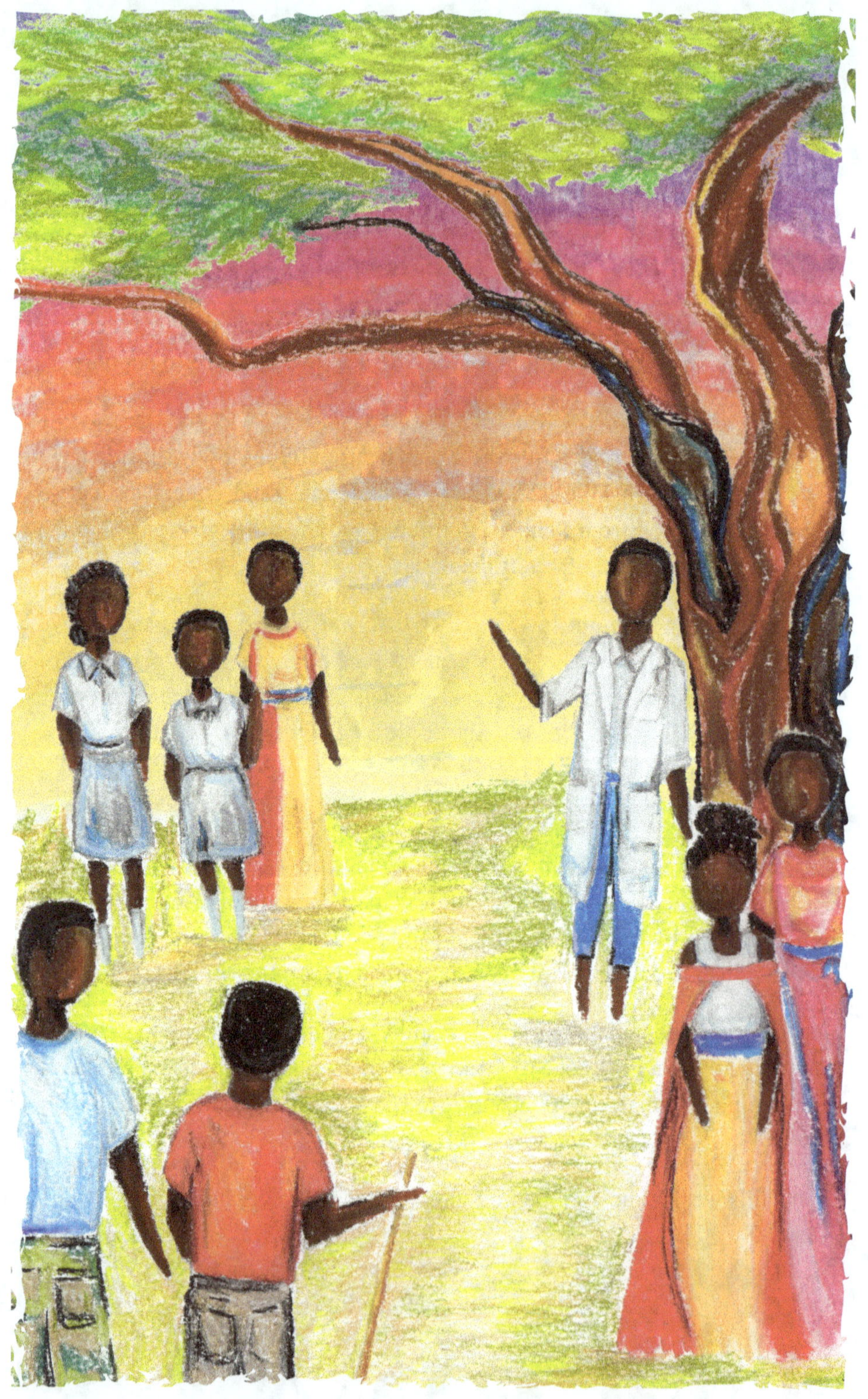

Chapter Seven

Maryam and Pendo strolled through the village, the warm sun casting a gentle glow on the vibrant surroundings. In the distance, the rhythmic sounds of laughter and the thud of a football reached their ears. Intrigued, they followed the lively echoes until they arrived at a makeshift football match where a group of young boys played.

Maryam nudged Pendo. "We need some support from the boys. If women are to step up and raise the level of beliefs about gender and abuse, they need some help!"

Pendo and Maryam knew they could never approach a whole group of boys. The struggle to show "manliness" would win out over sensibility.

"How would we ever get support from the boys?" Pendo thought out loud. Maryam gave a knowing glance to her cousin Kwame as the group of boys paused the game. Kwame and Maryam had grown up in their large extended family together. They had a special friendship that was rare between sexes. Through the years, Kwame had confided in Maryam how he wanted to protect his mother from the frequent beatings of his father. Maryam could only console but lately had been telling Kwame of the gatherings with Dr. Emma and how the support could possibly help his mother. Curious and nervous, Maryam and Pendo lingered nearby, overhearing bits of their conversation.

Kwame said, "Hey, I overheard these girls discussing topics being discussed by the new doctor at the clinic. You know, the one where they discuss important stuff under the acacia tree. She said they help with, you know, problems for women."

A hush fell over the group as the weight of Kwame's words settled in. Pendo exchanged a knowing look with Maryam, recognizing the significance of the moment. The reality of domestic challenges within their community was always there, though few dared to bring it to the forefront. However, the group of boys shrugged their shoulders and began playing again. Kwame gave Maryam a shoulder shrug and joined in the game once more.

Pendo sighed at the small accomplishment and quietly whispered to Maryam, "My whole life I would hear of so many of this village who suffer in abuse. Nobody should have to face these problems alone. There must be a solution. Do you feel it could ever be possible that we could talk about men respecting and protecting women?"

"All things are possible, Pendo, but it could take years, maybe decades. Don't you think?" Maryam answered herself as she thought aloud to Pendo. "The unspoken shame of abuse is so much a part of our culture. I think it will only stop when we as a new generation refuse to let it be part of our own future family."

"How do we do that? It seems to be just the way it is." Pendo straightened. "I hope my future husband understands that he is only as powerful as I am respected. Imagine what a happy life it is to be parents and good friends."

That week, the discussion group gathered again, with a more solemn tone and a few shy boys, including Kwame, joining the group. They were there from the strong encouragement of their head teacher. He had asked them to go and report back on any discussions they might need to continue within their class.

Dr. Emma, having spoken with the head teacher the previous week, was still pleasantly surprised to see them there. She gave a supportive smile and decided it was time to address the pressing issue of sexual safety and women's rights. As the boys sat in the back of the group, Dr. Emma began, her voice resonating with both compassion and determination. "Another grave concern for women in our village and around the world is their sexual safety and rights. Sadly, the choice to have consensual and respectful relationships is not always given. Many women have faced mistreatment and abuse or have been forced into situations against their will. This is a violation of their rights and an attempt to exert power over them. This happens to many girls as soon as they mature into women."

Dr. Emma changed to a lighter tone. "Let's hear from our younger girls. Tell us, girls, what kind of relationship would you like with your future husband?"

"Friendship."

"Safety and respect."

"Support and a helping hand."

"Strong and handsome."

"A good listener and patient."

"Respect and understanding of my cycle."

The aunties clapped, pleased at how far these young girls had come in the weeks since they had all started meeting.

Dr. Emma joined in. "All of these comments are wonderful attributes for some wonderful men. Imagine if all men could live up to these dreams. Unfortunately, some traditions do not honor the rights and safety of women. Girls' dreams are dashed when they grow up in a culture that places them below men in status. This issue is at the core of poverty and unhappiness in general in family life. Some women have been coerced into having sex for financial reasons, creating a cycle of poverty for her and the possible children that result from the coercion. Remember that every time sexual intercourse happens there is the possibility of a pregnancy. When a child is born outside the safety of a loving family, their health, happiness and well-being is greatly compromised. The impact of our cultural norms and the ongoing struggle for gender equality greatly affects sexual health."

Dr. Emma paused, allowing the weight of her words to sink in. She then spoke directly to the young girls, "When your sexual safety is threatened, it creates high-stress situations, making it difficult for you to thrive and be healthy sexually. Sexual abuse is a sad reality, but we, as women and concerned men, can work towards positive change in our culture concerning gender equality and women's safety."

Dr. Emma, with a somber yet determined expression, directed the conversation towards the profound consequences of sexual abuse. "No matter the age or relationship, unwanted sex causes harm to the body, mind, and spirit. It leaves individuals feeling

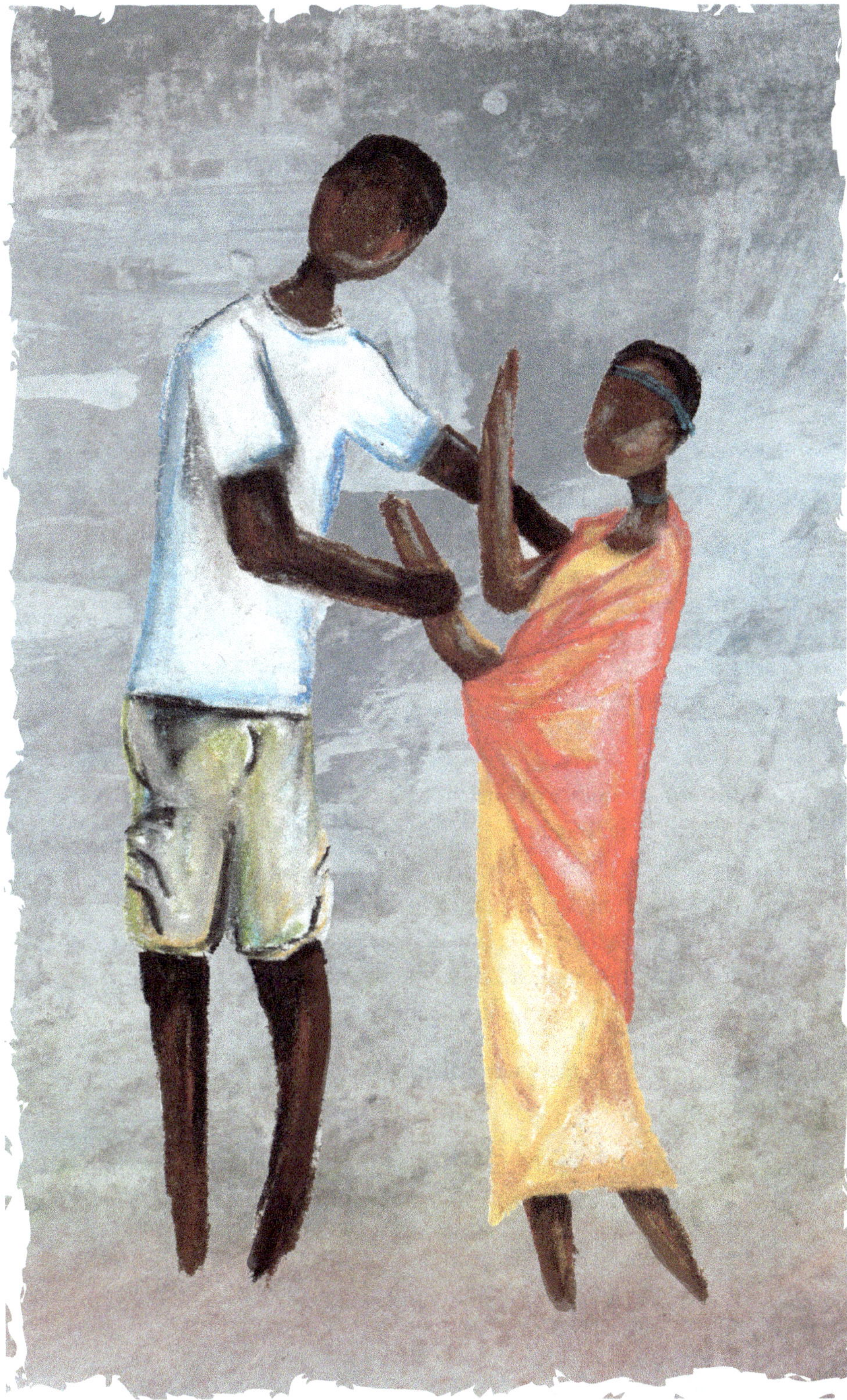

powerless, depressed, guilty, and ashamed. These heavy feelings can lead to a cycle of negative thoughts and behaviors."

To illustrate this point, Dr. Emma beckoned two older women from the gathering to share their experiences. One, with a downcast demeanor, spoke of life with an abusive husband, highlighting the relentless emotional turmoil and scars it left on her spirit. Kwame swallowed his deep sadness and empathy for this woman as he knew firsthand the anguish.

"I wake up each day with a weight on my chest," she said, her voice quivering. "The constant fear, the feeling of worthlessness… It was like living in a never-ending storm. I used to dream of love and happiness, but those dreams never came to be. I feel worthless and unlovable."

With a furrowed brow, Dr. Emma posed a question that hung in the air like a heavy cloud. "Is it too late for the women in the abusive situation?" She scanned the faces of the group.

Beside her, another woman, now free from the shackles of abuse, painted a different picture. Her eyes sparkled with a sense of self-worth. "I faced these same challenges, but I have found strength in God and within myself. I learned to stand tall, to show respect and not fear. I left that abusive situation and had to start at the bottom. But now, my days are filled with a different kind of peace. A peace that comes from knowing I am in control of my life."

Dr. Emma prompted her further, "Where can an abused woman seek help?"

"From the village elders, the support groups, and organizations that specialize in assisting survivors of abuse. Sharing experiences lightened my burden. I was reminded that I am not alone in my journey. I also formed a financial group, which created a safety net for me.”

Dr. Emma was so proud. “Education is a powerful tool. Acquiring skills empowers these women to stand on their own. It opens doors to financial independence, allowing them to shape their future in a healthy, happy, more holy way.”

“And lastly, embracing self-care is an act of reclaiming one’s well-being. Remembering that the healthy am I mantra starts with how we treat our bodies. Even if someone else is abusing us, we always control how we treat ourselves, how we talk to ourselves, and most importantly, it doesn’t affect how God feels about our holiness.”

“In the case of rape, what can be done in terms of prevention?” Dr. Emma asked.

Grace shyly raised her hand. “I have learned to be especially trusting of my instincts and be attuned to my surroundings. If a situation feels uncomfortable or unsafe, I leave immediately and I always try to have another friend, brother, or family member know where I am if I have to be alone.”

Dr. Emma added to her brave comment. “Keeping trusted friends, family members, or support groups informed about one’s whereabouts and concerns establishes a network of people ready to lend a helping hand. This network can serve as a protective shield. I’d bet these kind boys here today would be great shields of protection for the girls in this community.”

The boys shifted uncomfortably.

“Finally,” Dr. Emma concluded, “as humans, both men and women, we all want peace, safety, security and to be loved. How can we achieve this together?" She motioned towards the young men in the group to hear their opinions.

Grandma interjected, "It is a sad tradition we have here in Ubora Village that men dominate, and even "own" their wives. Many boys grow up seeing this and just repeat the pattern. The women grow up thinking they are property, especially if they are forced to marry at a young age. They know nothing of rights and have no legal help or even knowledge of legal help. It is an overwhelming and depressing problem!"

Dr. Emma reassured the group. "While it can be an overwhelming cultural barrier to this issue, we can start in small and simple ways. I would like to hear from our young men here today."

Kwame cleared his throat. "I do not know how to protect my mother. I sometimes fear she will be beaten to death. She doesn't feel as though she is valuable enough to even say it is wrong." His head rose. "I do know I want to be a good man, and show women that I can control my anger, not drink alcohol, and stay in control. I hope to have the courage to tell my family that I do not want a wife to be given to me. I want to choose her, and have her choose me. I want to be good friends with her and protect her and always have her feel safe with me."

"We can do better when we know better!" Maryam exclaimed.

Pendo added, "What if we all decide to change our tradition by supporting those being abused and standing up for everyone's dignity?"

The discussion group pledged to create an environment of support and understanding. Support would come by way of allowing all voices to be heard, even opinions and experiences that are difficult or different from their own. They also decided to discuss these issues openly in their own families and circles of friends and speak up when they see disrespect for women and talk of the consequences of such beliefs.

One of the aunties told a personal story of her abusive situation with a boyfriend when she was young. She spoke of the horror but also of some teachers who guided and strengthened her to end the relationship.

Farida and Nyah, sitting close together, listened with rapt attention. Farida, inspired by the stories and determined to make a difference, whispered to Nyah, "We need to be brave and share what we learn with our friends. It is time for change."

Just then, one of the boys, with a somber expression, raised his hand. "I need to share something," he said, his voice wavering. The group turned to him. "My sister, she has suffered her whole life because of the infections and bleeding that happened after going through FGM. She was so young, and it is tradition, but it changed her whole life, for the worse. I do not want any more girls to suffer like she did."

A profound silence enveloped the group. Dr. Emma approached the boy, placing a comforting hand on his shoulder. "Thank you for sharing your story. It takes great courage to speak out against such deeply rooted traditions. By sharing your sister's story, you honor her memory and help us all realize the urgency of our mission."

"Tell us more about your sister," Dr. Emma gently encouraged. "We need to understand the depth of this tragedy."

The boy, holding back tears, began to recount the ordeal, "My sister was only twelve. She was so full of life, always smiling and playing with her friends. One day, our parents told her that it was time for the ritual that would make her a woman. She was scared, but didn't want to disobey."

He paused, taking a deep breath before continuing, "The day came, and they took her to an elder woman's house. I wasn't allowed to go, but I could hear her screams from outside. It felt like an eternity before it stopped. When they brought her back, she was pale and in so much pain. They said it was normal, that she would heal…" He swallowed and looked away, fighting back the rush of tears. "But, she didn't. She had fevers and shakes and moaned in pain for weeks and then months. She stopped singing and even talking. She is a different person now, a sad and angry person."

Dr. Emma and the others listened with heavy hearts. Dr. Emma spoke softly, "Your sister's story is heartbreaking, but it also ignites a powerful call to action. We must work to end this harmful tradition and protect our girls. Her life, though short, can inspire change."

The group murmured in agreement, their resolve strengthening. One of the older boys, visibly moved, spoke up, "We can't let this continue. We need to educate our community about these dangers. We need to protect our sisters and daughters."

Kwame added, "We can start by talking to our friends and families, raising awareness. And we should support organizations that fight against FGM and provide medical care to those affected."

Dr. Emma nodded. "Education and awareness are crucial. We can also create safe spaces like this one for girls to talk about their fears and experiences. Let's empower them with knowledge and support."

The group discussed practical steps they could take, from organizing community meetings to creating informative pamphlets and collaborating with local leaders. They vowed to honor his sister's memory by working tirelessly to end FGM and promote the well-being of all girls in their village.

"Healthy am I, happy am I, holy am I." The group closed the meeting. Dr. Emma hugged each member and assured them that by being examples of this mantra, they could change their community, one person at a time.

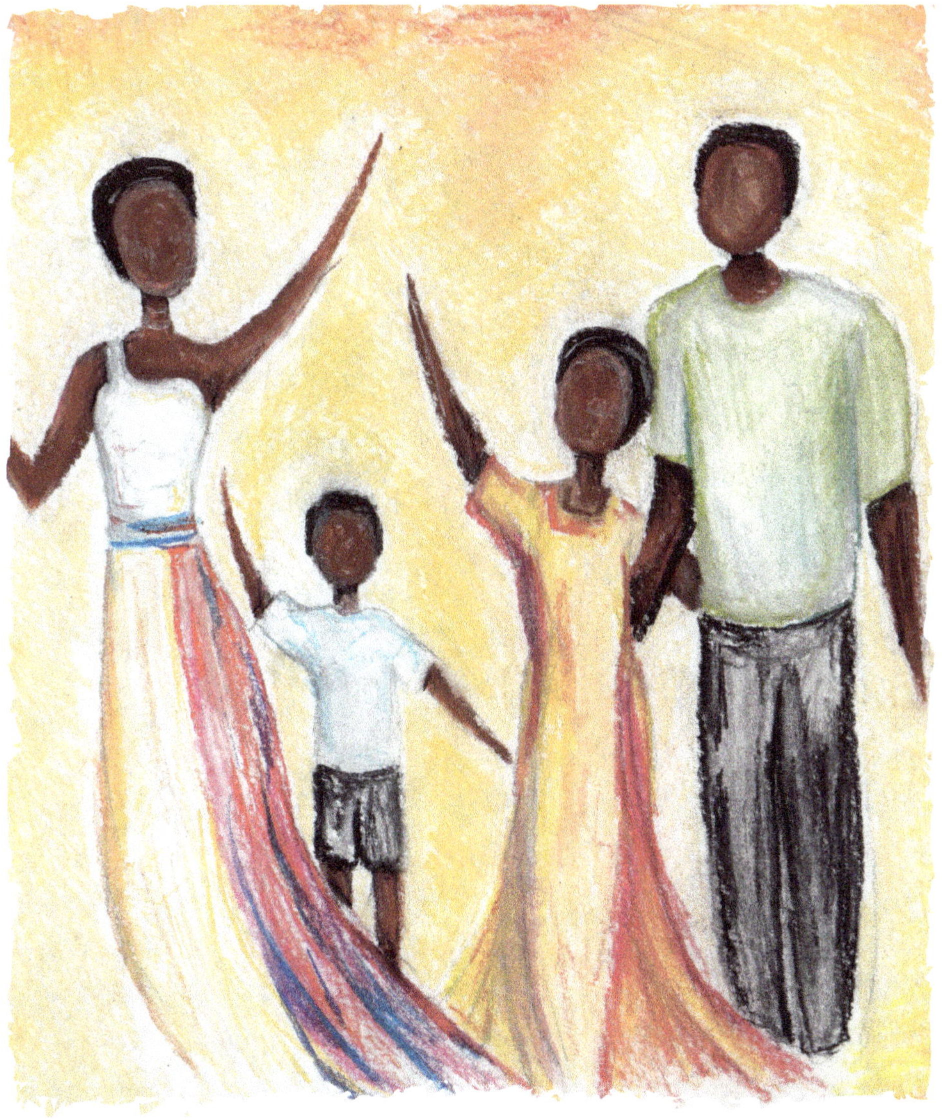

Chapter Eight

*P*endo, Maryam, Nyah, and Farida stayed to talk to Dr. Emma. Pendo spoke first, her eyes reflecting a mix of concern and resolve. "We've been thinking about the sexual abuse issue, and we believe it is time to shine a light on it. We want to create awareness, educate both girls and boys and work towards fostering an environment where everyone feels safe."

Maryam added, "We can't let any of these issues persist in the shadows. It is affecting the well-being of our fellow villagers, and it is time for a change."

Nyah, visibly troubled by the prospect of an impending early marriage, voiced her fears. "Dr. Emma, they call it tradition, but I am scared. I do not want my life to be decided for me."

Farida, who had experienced the physical and emotional pain of FGM firsthand, interjected firmly. "FGM is a violation of our rights and well-being. I want to challenge my family's beliefs and prevent other girls from going through what I endured."

Dr. Emma nodded, acknowledging the gravity of the situation. "You all have compassionate hearts and a sense of responsibility towards your community. Addressing such sensitive issues requires tact and empathy. How do you plan to approach this?"

Pendo outlined their preliminary plans. "We want to organize awareness sessions, maybe under the acacia tree or in the community center. We'll invite everyone—men, women, and the youth. We'll talk about the importance of consent, respect, and the consequences of sexual abuse. But we also want to create a safe space for survivors to come forward and seek support."

Maryam interjected, "Additionally, we thought of involving the local schools. Education is a powerful tool, and if we can instill these values early on, we might be able to prevent some of these issues."

Dr. Emma smiled, impressed by their thoughtful approach. "Education is indeed key. It is not just about raising awareness but also about changing mindsets. I'll support you in any way I can. If you need resources or guidance, consider me here."

Encouraged by Dr. Emma's support, they set out to organize their first awareness session. Pendo returned home from the village meeting. Her family was gathered in their modest living room and the atmosphere was tense. Her father, Ahmed, sat on one end of the room, while her older brother, Jamal, and her mother, Leila, sat on the other.

Ahmed, his brow furrowed with disapproval, spoke first. "Pendo, I heard you speak at the village meeting today. You know it is inappropriate for a young woman like you to speak about such topics publicly."

Pendo, her heart heavy with the impending confrontation, took a deep breath before responding. "Father, I only spoke because I believe it is an important issue that affects our community. Young girls are being forced into marriages that rob them of their futures. They are suffering, and I thought I could help raise awareness."

Jamal, equally disapproving, chimed in, "Pendo, you should know your place. These matters are not for girls to discuss openly. You're tarnishing our family's reputation by judging and shaming our tradition of allowing marriages, paying dowry, and arrangements between families."

Her mother joined in the scolding. "Pendo, we raised you to be modest and respectful. The elders in the village are very upset that you are stirring up such conversations."

Pendo's eyes welled with tears, but she could not back down. "I understand your concerns, but I could not ignore that this practice is not for the benefit of the girl, or her future family. Young girls are greatly endangered by abuse and early childbirth. I felt compelled to speak out."

Ahmed's frustration was evident as he stood up, his voice rising. "Pendo, you are not helping anyone by talking about these things. You're only bringing shame to our family. Who will listen to you?"

The room fell into an uncomfortable silence, tension thick in the air. She felt torn between her desire to make a difference and the expectations and disapproval of her family. The irony of her family's words felt heavy on her heart.

Her mother's expression was a mixture of disappointment and frustration. Her voice strained with a sense of betrayal. "Pendo, do you realize what you've done? You've embarrassed our family today with your outspokenness about those matters."

Pendo, tears still glistening in her eyes, mustered the courage to respond. "Mother, I didn't mean to embarrass anyone. I spoke because I wanted to help the girls in our village. They're suffering, don't you notice the problems with your friends who married too early?"

Leila's disappointment deepened as she shook her head. "Pendo, you do not understand. These topics are not for decent young women to decide. The choice is not ours. The arrangement of marriages is financial and often not abusive."

Despite her family's resistance, Pendo could not suppress the conviction that speaking out was the right thing to do. She took a deep breath. "Mother, I respect our traditions, but we cannot ignore the harm they cause."

Pendo decided it was time to share today's tragic story, hoping it would illustrate the gravity of the situation. She looked at her parents and brother, her voice steady but filled with emotion. "Let me tell you about Aisha, a girl from our neighboring village. She underwent FGM when she was just nine years old. The procedure was done in unsanitary conditions, and she suffered a severe infection. Aisha was in excruciating pain, but her cries were ignored because it was deemed normal."

Ahmed, visibly uncomfortable but trying to remain stoic, listened as she continued. "The infection spread, and Aisha became very ill. By the time her parents sought medical help, it was too late. She died a few weeks later from complications that could have been prevented. Aisha's death was a direct result of FGM."

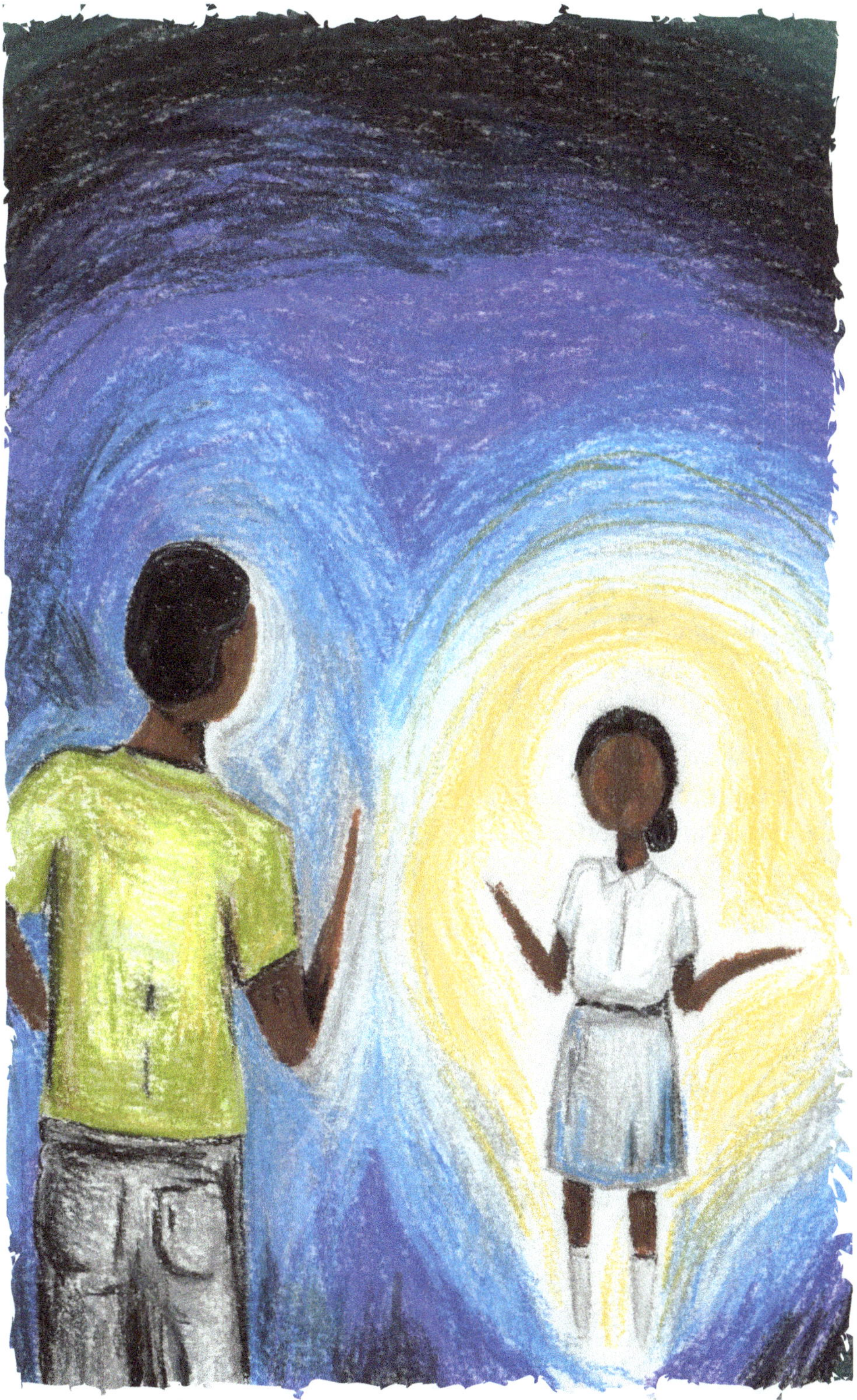

Leila's eyes filled with tears, and she clutched her hands tightly. Pendo pressed on, "Aisha's story is not unique. Many girls suffer in silence, their health and lives at risk because of this harmful practice. We must stop it. We must protect all the girls."

A heavy silence filled the room as the words sank in. Leila looked at Ahmed, her eyes pleading for understanding. "Ahmed, we can't ignore this. Our traditions should not come at the cost of our daughters' lives."

Ahmed's face hardened with resolve. "I understand your concerns, but our traditions define us. We cannot simply abandon them. Change takes time, and we must be cautious."

Jamal, who had been quietly listening, finally spoke up, his voice firm. "Father, Pendo is right. These practices are harming our community. We need to protect our girls, not endanger them. I am with them on this."

Ahmed glared at Jamal, clearly upset by his son's defiance. "Jamal, you should know better than to question our traditions. This is not your place."

Jamal's gaze didn't waver. "Father, it is our responsibility to question practices that harm our people. We can't turn a blind eye to the suffering."

Pendo, heartened by her brother's support, added softly, "Father, we are not asking to abandon all our traditions. We're asking to change the ones that hurt us. Please, think about it."

Ahmed stood up, his expression stern. "Enough. This discussion is over. We will uphold our traditions."

Pendo's heart sank at her father's words. She had hoped for support, understanding, or at least a glimmer of empathy. Instead, she felt like an outcast in her own family, torn between her desire to bring about change and the weight of tradition and family expectations.

As Ahmed left the room, Leila looked at her children with a mix of sorrow and pride. "Your father is stubborn, but maybe, just maybe, he will come to see the truth. Keep fighting for what's right. Change doesn't happen overnight."

Pendo and Jamal exchanged determined looks. They knew the path ahead would be difficult, but they were united in their resolve to protect the girls of their village and to challenge the traditions that brought harm. Pendo's bravery in sharing Aisha's story and Jamal's unexpected support gave them hope that change was possible, even if it required patience and persistence.

Pendo quietly helped her mother prepare dinner while silently repeating to herself, "Healthy am I, happy am I, holy am I." It brought peace to her heart as she vowed to honor both her family and herself. She wondered if she could take a kinder, gentler approach to helping facilitate change in her community.

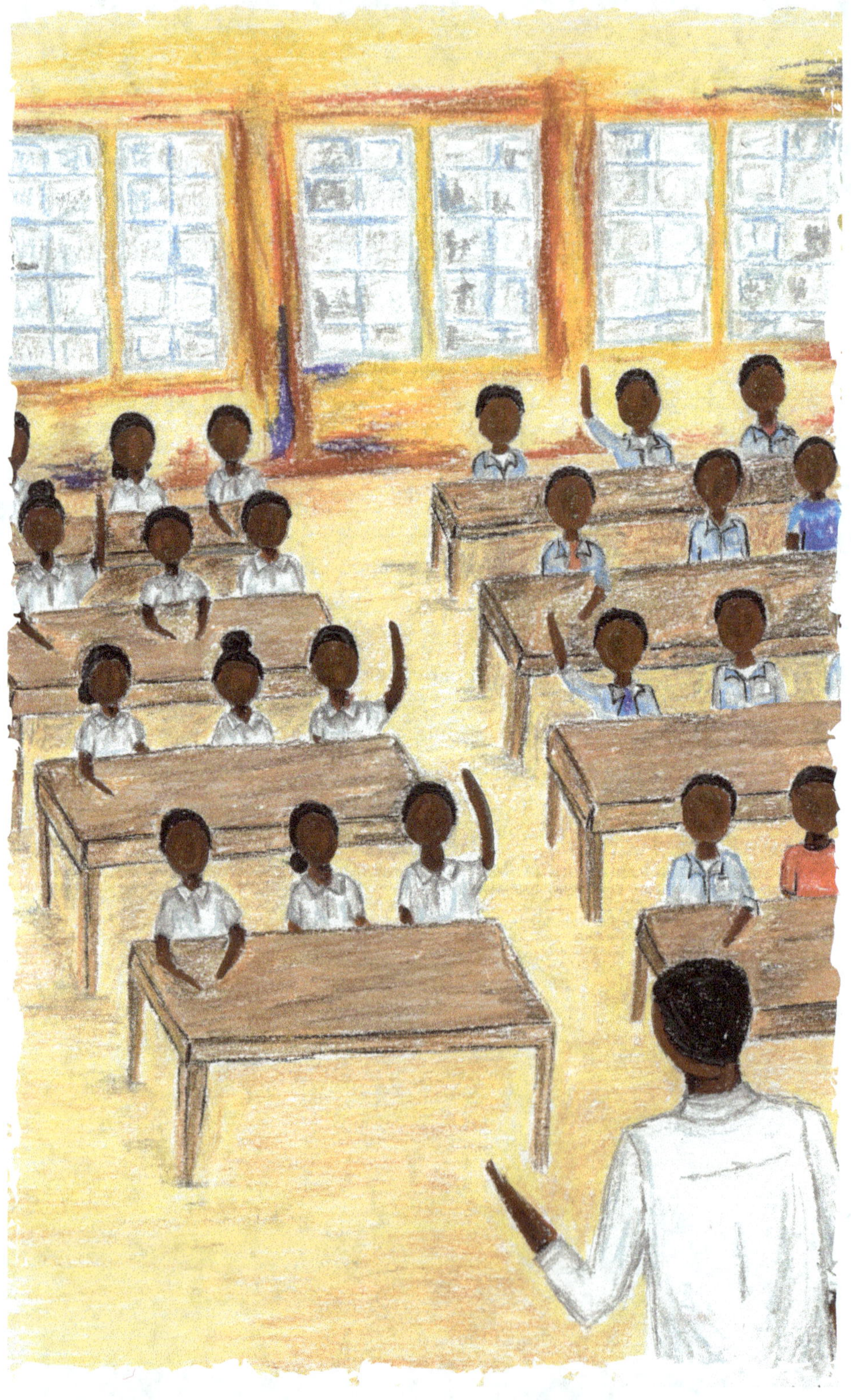

Chapter Nine

The next day, Pendo arrived at the village school. The scolding from her father still weighed on her, but she remained resolute in her commitment. As she walked through the school grounds, she noticed a group of football-playing boys and some male teachers huddled together.

One of the male teachers, who had a reputation for being outspoken, approached Pendo with a determined look in his eyes. "Pendo, we heard about what happened at the village meeting yesterday. We think it is great that you are standing up for women."

Pendo was taken aback by this teacher's words and the support he represented. "Thank you. I appreciate your understanding."

"The principal and I agreed we should support you in raising awareness about these issues. We want strong girls in our schools, in our community, and in our families. However, it is not our place to change to the whole of our society. Bias and opinion are very difficult to change and can take decades."

Jamal, Pendo's brother, happened to overhear the conversation. After challenging his father on these issues the previous day, he felt even more empowered to stand with his sister. Pendo's heart swelled with gratitude as she realized she had unexpected allies in her mission. Her teacher and principal's acknowledgment starkly contrasted the disapproval she had faced at home the previous evening. She thanked her teacher sincerely. Pendo imagined that one day soon she would have the courage to go and speak with the head teacher and discuss how they could improve the issues that plagued the girls in their school.

That day came sooner than expected. The principal met with Pendo and the head woman teacher. He expressed to them his concern that the graduation rate of females to males was not acceptable and encouraged them to talk with the teachers of the seventh and eighth-grade levels for ideas to improve this rate.

After that, Pendo was so pleased to see those teachers beneath the acacia tree. They grew in knowledge and appreciation for the female body. Dr. Emma helped them feel more confident in teaching the girls in their school. They discussed the many concerns they had for their student's safety and well-being along with the simple facts of the feminine cycle and how best to care for it. Pendo noticed a drastic improvement in the girls' confidence at school. They trusted their teachers more and felt more empowered to make healthy choices. A huge smile spread across Pendo's face as she passed by the seventh-grade girls' science lesson and they were each holding different colors of paper and repeating, **"Healthy am I, happy am I, holy am I."**

Later that year, Pendo, Maryam, Farida and Nyah were in shock as they were under the acacia tree with Dr. Emma. The teachers were explaining how much Dr. Emma's meetings were influencing the community as a whole. Barbara, the eighth-grade head teacher, filled them in on the good news. "The male teachers surprised the boys who came to the assembly to hear the winner of the science scores. Instead, they heard all about period poverty, FGM, and early forced marriages!" The women clapped and laughed in unison.

"The best part," Barbara continued, "was when he suggested that period poverty happens because of ignorance and apathy of the males. He even suggested that what starts with period poverty leads to other harms like FGM and early forced marriages, affecting the whole village. He further explained that to allow ridicule of girls is the same as not protecting their girls from sexual predators, Sugar Daddies, sexual taunting, risky sexual behavior, or abuse. He reminded them that the girls in their school were the future mothers and leaders of their own families and communities. He suggested that men were demeaning themselves by demeaning womanhood. He added that girls being sold or used as income in any way was a symptom of men not leading or stepping up to their full potential. He reminded everyone that men cannot rise while stepping on the women in their society."

Dr. Emma could not help but grab her heart in joy. "Oh my, this is the best news!"

"Some of the boys looked very ashamed, some of them scoffed," Barbara said. "I know many of these boys live in homes where the father beats his mother. So many of us see first-hand the effects of male domination in the family. They see what happens when the mother is overworked and lives in fear. I hope many of those boys felt the importance of supporting women, not ruling over them."

Dr. Emma looked to the group. "Well, how do we as women in the community support these efforts of the school?"

Barbara was quiet but firm, "I suggested to the principal that we start with small but important changes in our school community. The assembly speech was a very big milestone; however, I told him that it would be nice for the boys to discuss in detail how they can look around for girls in their school who might need extra protection from men when they walk long distances or fetch water. And at the very least, never to ridicule a girl who needs period supplies."

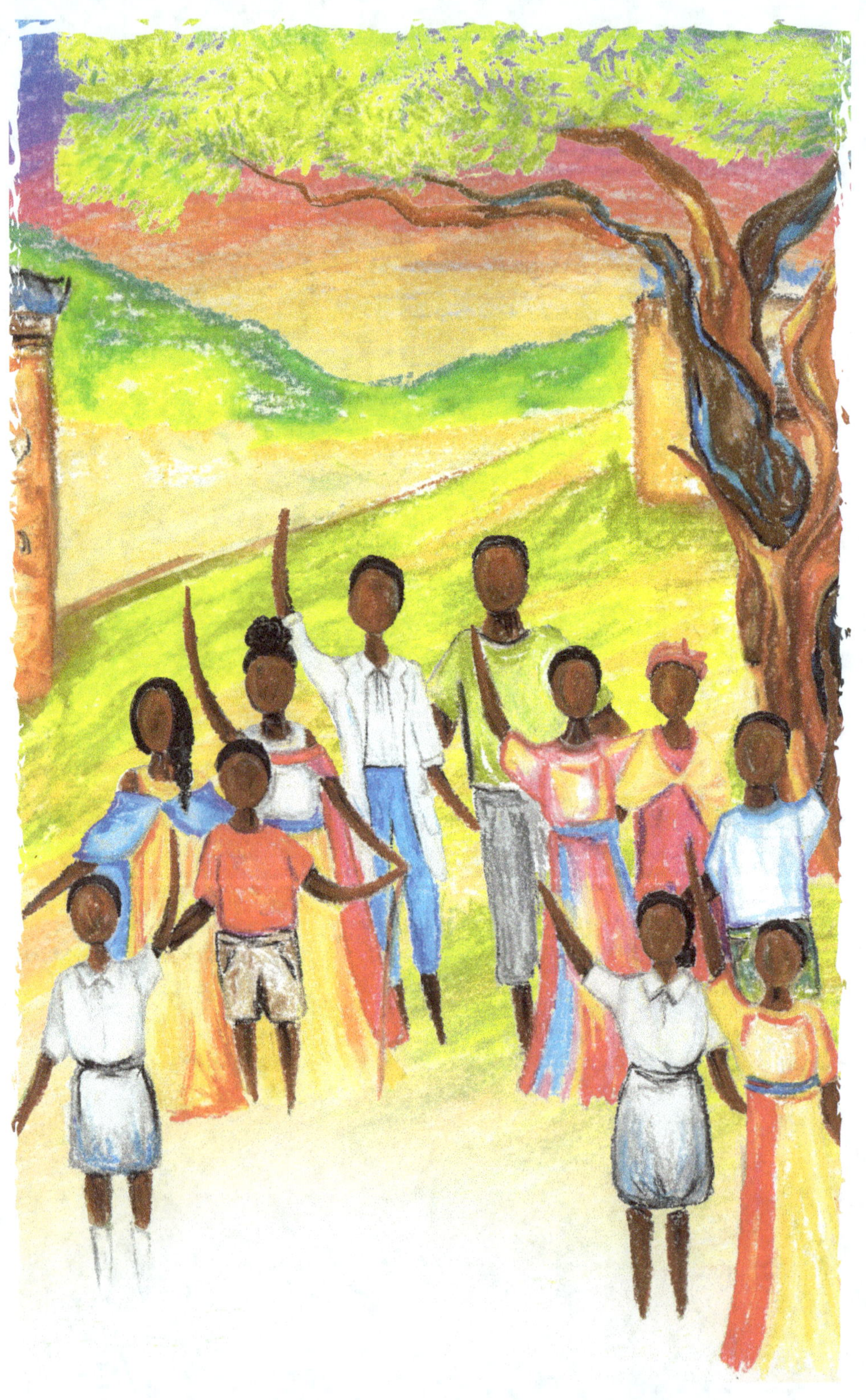

Chapter Ten

ONE YEAR LATER

While walking the dusty road home, Maryam grabbed Pendo's arm in excitement. "Can you believe it? It wasn't so long ago that you were wondering if you could ever go to school during your period. Now look at you. You are a superhero, Pendo!"

A shy smile of acknowledgment spread across Pendo's face. While she didn't feel like a superhero, she had found support from unexpected people. She knew that with the backing of teachers and the principal, she could continue her efforts to raise awareness about period poverty. "Oh Maryam, I still feel like a scared girl most of the time, but when I think of what could've happened to me without you and Dr. Emma...." Pendo's voice trailed.

Maryam turned to Pendo with a bright smile. "You know how much I have admired Dr. Emma and her work. Helping women and girls understand their health and power has become my passion, too."

Pendo nodded, understanding the depth of Maryam's aspirations. "Yes, you've always talked about wanting to make a difference like Dr. Emma does."

Maryam took a deep breath and shared her ambitious plan. "I have decided I want to graduate from high school and follow in Dr. Emma's footsteps to medical school."

Pendo's eyes widened with excitement. "That is incredible! But you know that is a long and challenging journey. Medical school is not easy to get into or pay for."

Maryam's determination shone through as she replied, "I know it won't be easy, but I can't just stand by."

Pendo could not help but feel inspired by her friend's dedication. "I believe in you. You've always been the risk-taker, and I know you'll achieve your dream. Dr. Emma will be proud to have you following in her footsteps."

Maryam smiled, a glimmer of hope in her eyes. "Thank you. With Dr. Emma's guidance and the backing of friends like you, I'll give it my all. This journey will begin with the difficult conversations that you are committed to continuing in our village. You will be my best support."

Dr. Emma was pleased with the steadily increasing size of the crowd. Each week, her words were a beacon of hope amid shadows that had plagued Ubora Village. "Silence only strengthens the chains of abuse and shame. We must be brave, for ourselves and the generations that will follow. Together, we can create a village where every voice is heard, no one lives in fear, and the light of knowledge and empowerment dispels the shadows of the past."

Pendo could not help but think about her family's initial disapproval and the shame associated with her desire to speak out about violence towards women and child marriage. It was a painful reminder of how deeply ingrained these issues were in their village. Thank goodness her brother and parents had finally lent their support.

Dr. Emma continued, "Remember, my dear ones, it is not just about speaking out against the shadows but also supporting one another. We are a community, and we can be a force for change. Let us stand with those who have suffered in silence, extend our hands to those in need, and be the light that guides our village towards a brighter future."

As Dr. Emma concluded her impassioned speech, the atmosphere under the acacia tree was charged with a sense of determination. Inspired by her words, the crowd felt a newfound strength welling up within them. Pendo and Maryam could see that it wasn't about just the two of them and their bravery, but they could rely on each person there. Each person had a unique voice and a unique circle of influence.

Boys and men from the village had become supporters and protectors of the women and girls. They were sprinkled throughout the audience. All the voices came together to close the week's session. **"Healthy are we, happy are we, holy are we."** The words were solidarity, bridging the gap between different perspectives and genders.

Among the crowd, Farida and Nyah listened intently. Farida had made significant progress over the year, becoming a vocal advocate against FGM. She had even convinced her family of the dangers, sharing Aisha's harrowing story of complications from FGM. Nyah, who had faced the threat of early marriage, now stood strong, supported by her newfound friends and teachers.

As the meeting concluded, Farida approached Pendo and Maryam. "I can't believe how far we've come," she said, her voice filled with pride. "A year ago, I could not have imagined standing here, speaking out against FGM and supporting other girls."

Nyah nodded in agreement. "And I never thought I'd escape an early marriage. Thanks to all of you, I plan to finish school and maybe even go to college."

Pendo smiled, feeling a deep sense of fulfillment. "We've all come a long way, and we still have a long way to go. But together, we are making a difference." The graduation rate for girls had improved significantly, and the school environment had become more supportive and empowering for female students.

Maryam added, "And it is not just us. Look at how the whole village is starting to change. Our voices are being heard, and we are stronger together."

Pendo's father, Ahmed, who had been initially resistant to change, finally approached the group. His face was thoughtful, and he seemed to struggle with his words. "Pendo, I have been thinking a lot. Maybe... maybe there is some truth in what you and your friends have been saying. I still hold our traditions dear, but I can't ignore the harm they've caused. Perhaps it is time we looked at things differently."

Pendo's heart swelled with hope. Her brother Jamal, who had quietly supported her all along, stepped forward and put a hand on their father's shoulder. "Father, it is not about abandoning our traditions but evolving them to protect and uplift everyone in our community."

Ahmed nodded slowly. "Yes, you are right, Jamal. It is time we became ambassadors for change."

90

As the sun set behind the acacia tree, casting long shadows over the gathered villagers, Pendo, Maryam, Farida, and Nyah felt a deep sense of unity and purpose. They had started a movement that was not only changing their village but also inspiring neighboring communities. They knew the journey ahead was long and fraught with challenges, but with each other's support and the growing backing of their community, they were ready to face whatever came next.

The collaborative spirit of the village, encompassing both boys and girls, was rising together as catalysts for change. The unity despite disagreement displayed in addressing some of the most difficult challenges sent ripples through the entire community.

The newfound solidarity soon extended beyond the village borders, inspiring neighboring communities to initiate similar conversations. The collective efforts of their village became a beacon of hope and resilience, echoing far beyond its immediate surroundings. And those echoes reverberated.

Healthy are WE.

Happy are WE.

Holy are WE.